D1483089

Cartilage Injuries in the Pediatric Knee

Guest Editors

HARPAL K. GAHUNIA, MSc, PhD
PAUL S. BABYN, MDCM, FRCPC

ORTHOPEDIC CLINICS OF NORTH AMERICA

www.orthopedic.theclinics.com

April 2012 • Volume 43 • Number 2

SAUNDERS an imprint of ELSEVIER, Inc.

W.B. SAUNDERS COMPANY
A Division of Elsevier Inc.

1600 John F. Kennedy Blvd. ● Suite 1800 ● Philadelphia, PA 19103-2899.

http://www.orthopedic.theclinics.com

ORTHOPEDIC CLINICS OF NORTH AMERICA Volume 43, Number 2
April 2012 ISSN 0030-5898, ISBN-13: 978-1-4557-3905-9

Editor: David Parsons

Orthopedic Clinics of North America (ISSN 0030-5898) is published quarterly by Elsevier Inc., 360 Park Avenue South, New York, NY 10010-1710. Months of issue are January, April, July, and October. Business and Editorial Offices: 1600 John F. Kennedy Blvd., Suite 1800, Philadelphia, PA 19103-2899. Customer Service Office: 3251 Riverport Lane, Maryland Heights, MO 63043. Periodicals postage paid at New York, NY and additional mailing offices. Subscription prices are $293.00 per year for (US individuals), $554.00 per year for (US institutions), $347.00 per year (Canadian individuals), $664.00 per year (Canadian institutions), $427.00 per year (international individuals), $664.00 per year (international institutions), $144.00 per year (US students), $208.00 per year (Canadian and international students). Foreign air speed delivery is included in all *Clinics* subscription prices. All prices are subject to change without notice. **POSTMASTER:** Send change of address to *Orthopedic Clinics of North America*, **Elsevier Health Sciences Division, Subscription Customer Service, 3251 Riverport Lane, Maryland Heights, MO 63043. Customer Service (orders, claims, online, change of address): Elsevier Health Sciences Division, Subscription Customer Service, 3251 Riverport Lane, Maryland Heights, MO 63043. Tel: 1-800-654-2452 (U.S. and Canada); 314-447-8871 (outside U.S. and Canada). Fax: 314-447-8029. E-mail: journalscustomerservice-usa@elsevier. com (for print support); journalsonlinesupport-usa@elsevier.com (for online support).**

Reprints. For copies of 100 or more, of articles in this publication, please contact the Commercial Reprints Department, Elsevier Inc., 360 Park Avenue South, New York, NY 10010-1710. Tel.: 212-633-3812; Fax: 212-462-1935; E-mail: reprints@elsevier.com.

Orthopedic Clinics of North America is covered in *MEDLINE/PubMed* (*Index Medicus*), *Cinahl, Excerpta Medica,* and *Cumulative Index to Nursing and Allied Health Literature.*

Printed in the United States of America.

Contributors

GUEST EDITOR

HARPAL K. GAHUNIA, MSc, PhD
President and CEO, Orthopedic Science
Consulting Services, Oakville, Ontario, Canada

AUTHORS

HIROSHI ASAHARA, MD, PhD
Department of Molecular and Experimental
Medicine, Scripps Research Institute,
La Jolla, California

MILVA BATTAGLIA, MD
Department of Radiology, Rizzoli Orthopaedic
Institute, Bologna, Italy

ROBERTO BUDA, MD
II Clinic of Orthopaedics and Traumatology,
Rizzoli Orthopaedic Institute, Bologna, Italy

WILLIAM D. BUGBEE, MD
Division of Orthopedic Surgery, Scripps Clinic,
La Jolla, California

KIZHER S. BUHARY, MD, BE
Division of Paediatric Orthopaedics, National
University Hospital; Medical Student, Duke-
NUS Graduate Medical School, Singapore

MARCO CAVALLO, MD
II Clinic of Orthopaedics and Traumatology,
Rizzoli Orthopaedic Institute, Bologna, Italy

ELAINE F. CHAN, MS
Department of Bioengineering, University
of California, San Diego, San Diego, California

**ASHWIN CHOWDHARY, MBBS, D Orth,
MS Orth, MRCS**
Clinical Fellow, Division of Paediatric
Orthopaedics, National University Hospital,
Singapore

GARY S. FIRESTEIN, MD
Department of Medicine, University of
California, San Diego, San Diego, California

HARPAL K. GAHUNIA, MSc, PhD
President and CEO, Orthopedic Science
Consulting Services, Oakville, Ontario,
Canada

SANDRO GIANNINI, MD
II Clinic of Orthopaedics and Traumatology,
Rizzoli Orthopaedic Institute, Bologna, Italy

DANIEL A. GRANDE, PhD
Department of Orthopaedics, Feinstein
Institute for Medical Research, North-Shore
Long Island Jewish Medical Center,
Manhasset, New York

RICKY HARJANTO, BS
Department of Bioengineering, University
of California, San Diego, San Diego,
California

HARISH S. HOSALKAR, MD
Department of Orthopedic Surgery, Rady
Children's Hospital, San Diego, California

JAMES H.P. HUI, MBBS, FRCS, MD
Associate Professor and Head, Division
of Paediatric Orthopaedics, National University
Hospital, Singapore

NOZOMU INOUE, MD, PhD
Department of Biomedical Engineering,
Doshisha University, Kyoto, Japan;
Department of Orthopedic Surgery, Rush
University Medical Center, Chicago, Illinois

DENNIS E. KRAMER, MD
Instructor, Division of Sports Medicine,
Department of Orthopaedic Surgery,
Children's Hospital Boston, Harvard Medical
School, Boston, Massachusetts

THOMAS F. LAPORTA, MD
Department of Orthopaedics, Long Island
Jewish Medical Center, New Hyde Park,
New York

FACUNDO LAS HERAS, MD, PhD
Assistant Professor of Pathology, University
of Chile Clinical Hospital, University of Chile,
Santiago, Chile

EDWARD Y. LEE, MD, MPH
Department of Radiology, Children's Hospital
Boston and Harvard Medical School, Boston,
Massachusetts

MARTIN K. LOTZ, MD
Department of Molecular and Experimental
Medicine, Scripps Research Institute,
La Jolla, California

KOICHI MASUDA, MD
Department of Orthopedic Surgery, University
of California, San Diego, San Diego, California

AIDEN MOKTASSI, MD, FRCPC
Lecturer, Department of Medical Imaging,
Mount Sinai Hospital, University of Toronto,
Toronto, Ontario, Canada

M. LUCAS MURNAGHAN, MD, MEd, FRCSC
Assistant Professor, Division of Orthopaedic
Surgery, Department of Surgery, The Hospital
for Sick Children, University of Toronto,
Toronto, Ontario, Canada

J. LEE PACE, MD
Fellow, Division of Sports Medicine,
Department of Orthopaedic Surgery,
Children's Hospital Boston, Harvard Medical
School, Boston, Massachusetts

CHARLES A. POPKIN, MD
Clinical Fellow, Division of Orthopaedic
Surgery, The Hospital for Sick Children,
University of Toronto, Toronto, Ontario,
Canada

KENNETH P.H. PRITZKER, MD, FRCPC
Professor, Department of Laboratory Medicine
and Pathobiology; Professor, Department of
Surgery, University of Toronto; Pathologist,
Pathology and Laboratory Medicine, Mount
Sinai Hospital, Toronto, Ontario, Canada

RICARDO RESTREPO, MD
Department of Radiology, Miami Children's
Hospital, Miami, Florida

ALEXANDER RICHTER, MD, MS
Department of Orthopaedics, North-Shore
Long Island Jewish Medical Center,
Manhasset, New York

ROBERT L. SAH, MD, ScD
Department of Bioengineering; Institute
of Engineering in Medicine, University
of California, San Diego, San Diego, California

NICHOLAS A. SGAGLIONE, MD
Department of Orthopaedics, North-Shore
Long Island Jewish Medical Center, University
Orthopaedic Associates, Great Neck,
New York

FRANCESCA VANNINI, MD, PhD
II Clinic of Orthopaedics and Traumatology,
Rizzoli Orthopaedic Institute, Bologna, Italy

LAWRENCE M. WHITE, MD, FRCPC
Professor, Department of Medical Imaging,
Mount Sinai Hospital, University of Toronto,
Toronto, Ontario, Canada

Contents

Articular Cartilage Development: A Molecular Perspective   155

Facundo Las Heras, Harpal K. Gahunia, and Kenneth P.H. Pritzker

> In this article, development of articular cartilage and endochondral ossification is reviewed, from the perspective of both morphologic aspects of histogenesis and molecular biology, particularly with respect to key signaling molecules and extracellular matrix components most active in cartilage development. The current understanding of the roles of transforming growth factor β and associated signaling molecules, bone morphogenic proteins, and molecules of the Wnt-β catenin system in chondrogenesis are described. Articular cartilage development is a highly conserved complex biological process that is dynamic and robust in nature, which proceeds well without incident or failure in all joints of most young growing individuals.

Structural and Functional Maturation of Distal Femoral Cartilage and Bone During Postnatal Development and Growth in Humans and Mice   173

Elaine F. Chan, Ricky Harjanto, Hiroshi Asahara, Nozomu Inoue, Koichi Masuda, William D. Bugbee, Gary S. Firestein, Harish S. Hosalkar, Martin K. Lotz, and Robert L. Sah

> The size and shape of joints markedly affect their biomechanical properties, but the macroscopic 3-dimensional (3-D) mechanism and extent of cartilage and joint maturation during normal growth are largely unknown. This study qualitatively illustrates the development of the bone-cartilage interface in the knee during postnatal growth in humans and C57BL/6 wild-type mice, quantitatively defines the 3-D shape using statistical shape modeling, and assesses growth strain rates in the mouse distal femur. Accurate quantification of the cartilage-bone interface geometry is imperative for furthering the understanding of the macroscopic mechanisms of cartilage maturation and overall joint development.

Effect of Exercise on Articular Cartilage   187

Harpal K. Gahunia and Kenneth P.H. Pritzker

> This review primarily focuses on how the macromolecular composition and architecture of articular cartilage and its unique biomechanical properties play a pivotal role in the ability of articular cartilage to withstand mechanical loads several magnitudes higher than the weight of the individual. Current findings on short-term and long-term effects of exercise on human articular cartilage are reviewed, and the importance of appropriate exercises for individuals with normal and diseased or aberrated cartilage is discussed.

Imaging of Osteochondritis Dissecans   201

Aiden Moktassi, Charles A. Popkin, Lawrence M. White, and M. Lucas Murnaghan

> Osteochondritis dissecans (OCD) is a localized process that affects the subchondral bone and can progress to the overlying articular cartilage. The cause of this lesion remains elusive. With the vague clinical symptoms and signs of OCD, imaging plays

a vital role in making the diagnosis and helping with the prognosis of OCD lesions. This article reviews current imaging modalities for the assessment of OCD including conventional radiography, nuclear medicine, computed tomography (CT), CT arthrography, magnetic resonance (MR) and MR arthrography. The role of imaging in evaluating healing of the OCD and articular congruity after surgical and nonsurgical management is discussed.

Juvenile idiopathic arthritis is a broad term used to describe a series of chronic arthritis occurring in children younger than 16 years of age. Even though the cause is not fully understood, several clues regarding the pathogenesis have been found. Diagnosis of the different types of juvenile idiopathic arthritis is made clinically, and imaging plays a role in answering specific questions pertaining to disease classification, staging, and outcome of treatment options.

Adolescents are predisposed to osteochondral (OC) injuries in the knee. The medial facet of the patella, the femoral trochlea, and the lateral femoral condyle are the most common sites of injury. Most of these injuries are classically traumatic but noncontact injuries. Surgery is warranted in most cases of OC fracture. Depending on size, condition, and location of the lesion, options include OC fragment reduction and internal fixation or excision and cartilage resurfacing. Understanding of how to diagnose and treat OC fractures will help optimize outcomes.

Osteochondritis dissecans (OCD) is an increasingly common cause of knee pain and dysfunction among skeletally immature and young adult patients. An ideal treatment strategy with an optimal surgical technique to repair the osteochondral lesions in these patients is still controversial. The goal of this study is to evaluate and report the clinical and MRI findings for the treatment of OCD in the pediatric knee with bone marrow–derived cell transplantation by using a one-step surgical technique.

The repair of articular cartilage defects in patients' knees presents a particular challenge to the orthopedic surgeon because cartilage lacks the ability to repair or regenerate itself. Various cartilage repair techniques have not produced a superior or uniform outcome, which has led to a new generation of cartilage repair based on tissue-engineering strategies and the use of biological scaffolds. Clinical advances have been made regarding the regeneration of articular cartilage, and continue to be made toward the achievement of a suitable treatment method for resurfacing osteochondral defects, through cartilage tissue engineering and the use of pluripotent cells seeded on bio-scaffolds.

James H.P. Hui, Kizher S. Buhary, and Ashwin Chowdhary

The treatment of articular cartilage lesions is complicated, but novel tissue engineering approaches seem to improve the outcome. A tissue engineering approach is less invasive and reduces surgical time, periosteal hypertrophy, and morbidity. Cell-based therapies using scaffolds have advantages compared with microfracture techniques, but the efficacy and cost-effectiveness need to be investigated. Second-generation cell-based therapies have lower morbidity and the ease of the technique is not significantly different from that of first-generation autologous chondrocyte implantation techniques. Third-generation cell-based therapies such as the use of tissue engineered scaffolds need to be studied in more detail.

Orthopedic Clinics of North America

THE CLINICS ARE NOW AVAILABLE ONLINE!

Access your subscription at:
www.theclinics.com

Preface

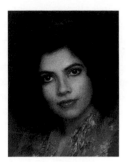

Harpal K. Gahunia, MSc, PhD
Guest Editor

The April 2012 issue of the *Orthopedic Clinics of North America* focuses on the various aspects of cartilage in the pediatric knee. Articular cartilage is a dynamic, robust, and complex tissue that intrigues as well as perplexes many who are interested in this field. The knee is one of the joints most commonly injured during sport-related activities in children. Articular cartilage in children is a highly organized structure with an extracellular matrix containing varying concentrations of macro- and micromolecules, which repeatedly undergo resorption and formation while maintaining the shape of the joint throughout growth. Injury to any part of this complex system can disrupt the functional properties of cartilage, which may lead to further joint degeneration. Although articular cartilage has intrinsic capacity for repair and regeneration, the organized structure of immature cartilage is particularly difficult to restore or duplicate once it is damaged or lost. The purpose of this issue is to gain a basic understanding of articular cartilage biology in children in terms of normal structure and function during the various stages of development and growth, and to integrate that knowledge with the clinical aspects of diagnosis and treatment of diseased or injured cartilage.

This issue encompasses a broad number of disciplines and several review topics related to young articular cartilage. The basic biology of immature articular cartilage including its structure and function with emphasis on molecular biology during various stages of development is presented by Las Heras, Gahunia, and Pritzker. The macromolecular composition and architecture of articular cartilage and its unique biomechanical properties play a pivotal role in the ability of articular cartilage

to withstand mechanical loads. The development of cartilage–bone interface in the knee during postnatal growth in humans and wild-type mice is presented in detail by Chan, Harjanto, Asahara, Inoue, Masuda, Bugbee, Firestein, Hosalkar, Lotz, and Sah. The impact of exercise on knee articular cartilage and appropriate exercises for individuals with normal or diseased cartilage are discussed by Gahunia and Pritzker. Magnetic resonance imaging plays an important role in the early diagnosis of diseased/injured cartilage, planning treatment, and the posttreatment follow-up to determine the success of surgical interventions. Excellent reviews on the epidemiology, pathogenesis, and magnetic resonance imaging of osteochondritis dessicans is presented by Moktassi, Popkin, White, and Murnaghan and of arthritis in children is presented by Restrepo and Lee. The repair of osteochondral lesions in the knee presents a challenge to the orthopaedic surgeons, in particular, treating young, active individuals. Kramer and Pace describe the acute traumatic and sports-related osteochondral injuries and treatment strategies for knee cartilage repair. Vannini, Battaglia, Buda, Cavallo, and Giannini describe an innovative "one-step" surgical strategy with bone marrow derived cell transplantation for the treatment of osteochondral lesions in the pediatric knee. The latest trend in cartilage engineering strategies is the use of biocompatible, biodegradable, and structurally as well as mechanically stable scaffolds that can allow successful loading of appropriate cells and the infiltration and attachment of appropriate bioactive molecules. These topics are reviewed in detail by LaPorta, Richter, Sgaglione, and Grande, and also by Hui, Buhary, and Chowdhary.

Orthop Clin N Am 43 (2012) ix–x
doi:10.1016/j.ocl.2012.03.002

Attempting to highlight the complexities of cartilage repair is a daunting task. I am much indebted to the authors for their thoughtful and scholarly input. It is wonderful to have contributions from worldwide leaders in the fields of orthopedic surgery, radiology, pathology, epidemiology, rehabilitation science, basic science, and cartilage engineering who came together to offer their invaluable insights toward this very complex topic of immature articular cartilage in health, disease, diagnosis, and healing. Through their dedication and highly collaborative efforts, they have made this outstanding issue possible.

I extend my sincere gratitude to the journal's managing editor, David Parsons, for his great enthusiasm and tremendous support of this issue. It was such a pleasure to work with him. Also, I am very thankful to David's staff for all their hard work and patience in ensuring the success and timely publication of this issue.

I envisage that this issue will stimulate scientific research and the exchange of knowledge and ideas among physicians, scientists, and researchers of the industry with an active interest in the field of immature cartilage biology, diagnosis of joint diseases, and repair treatments. The translation of clinical and basic sciences to health care and clinical practice will ultimately lead to the development of more effective treatment strategies for children afflicted by joint disorders.

Harpal K. Gahunia, MSc, PhD
Orthopedic Science Consulting Services
Oakville, Ontario, Canada

E-mail address:
harpal.gahunia@utoronto.ca

Articular Cartilage Development: A Molecular Perspective

Facundo Las Heras, MD, PhD[a],*,
Harpal K. Gahunia, MSc, PhD[b],
Kenneth P.H. Pritzker, MD, FRCPC[c,d,e]

KEYWORDS
- Articular cartilage • Epiphyseal cartilage
- Endochondral ossification

The histologic sequence in the formation of epiphyseal and articular cartilage is very familiar to every orthopedic surgeon. Accordingly, this article addresses the recent advances in molecular biology that are illuminating the factors that drive and control articular cartilage growth and development.

STRUCTURE AND FUNCTION OF ARTICULAR CARTILAGE

Articular cartilage, also referred to as hyaline cartilage, is a highly specialized connective tissue with biophysical properties consistent with its ability to withstand high compressive forces. Articular cartilage is termed hyaline because of its amorphous glassy appearance (**Fig. 1**) reflecting isotropic collagen distribution and abundant proteoglycan content. Its smooth, wear-resistant lubricated surface allows the bones to glide over one another with minimal friction and to absorb impact forces. The synovial fluid plays an important role in joint lubrication.[1] Adult cartilage is typically avascular, alymphatic, and aneural.[2] Nourishment is primarily provided through long-range diffusion of the synovial fluid.[3] Immature cartilage is in proximity to blood vessels; therefore, cartilage nourishment is also provided through diffusion of nutrients from blood. In addition, cartilage canals that connect the fetal and neonatal cartilage and subchondral bone are thought to contribute to the nourishment of cartilage. During growth and development, these cartilage canals extend as branches of the blood vessels to the articular-epiphyseal cartilage that forms the articulating surface of the bone, epiphyseal center of ossification, and growth plates.[4,5] Cartilage canals composed of blood vessels are seen in fetal articular cartilage. Postnatally, through the first year the cartilage canal distribution decreases and disappears.[4]

Articular cartilage is composed of an extracellular matrix with a complex macromolecular organization of predominantly collagen type II bundles intertwined with noncollagenous proteins, ions (primarily Na^+ and Cl^- ions), and soluble negatively charged proteoglycans molecules. Collagen type II, and proteoglycans account for 15% to 22% and 4% to 7% of the cartilage wet weight, respectively.[6]

The tissue fluid accounts for 65% to 80% of the wet weight of articular cartilage. This high fluid content enables nutrients and oxygen to diffuse through the cartilage matrix to its cells. Cartilage cells are composed of a single type termed chondrocytes, which are sparse in normal adult

---

The authors have no conflicts of interest to disclose.
[a] University of Chile Clinical Hospital, University of Chile, 999 Santos Dumont Avenue, Santiago, Chile
[b] Orthopedic Science Consulting Services, Oakville, Ontario, Canada
[c] Department of Laboratory Medicine & Pathobiology, University of Toronto, Toronto, Ontario, Canada
[d] Department of Surgery, University of Toronto, Toronto, Ontario, Canada
[e] Pathology & Laboratory Medicine, Mount Sinai Hospital, 600 University Avenue, Toronto, Ontario M5G 1X5, Canada
* Corresponding author.
E-mail address: facundo.lasheras@utoronto.ca

Orthop Clin N Am 43 (2012) 155–171
doi:10.1016/j.ocl.2012.01.003
0030-5898/12/$ – see front matter © 2012 Elsevier Inc. All rights reserved.

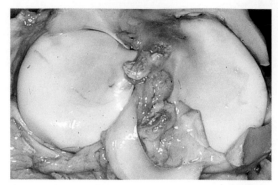

Fig. 1. Human tibial plateau showing amorphous glassy appearance of normal mature hyaline cartilage surface.

articular cartilage, accounting for less than 5% of the tissue wet weight.[7] By contrast, immature cartilage is highly cellular and the cellularity decreases with the maturation. Chondrocytes are responsible for generating and maintaining the cartilaginous extracellular environment.[8,9]

Collagen type II provides tensile strength to the cartilaginous matrix, and is important for the establishment of temporal and spatial organization with other matrix components such as the predominant proteoglycan termed aggrecan. Aggrecan is a composite macromolecule containing heavily sulfated glycosaminoglycans, which attract water molecules and forms large aggregates in cartilage. Aggrecan and other proteoglycans provide the cushioning capacity to the matrix, and also act to immobilize and store growth factors, thereby functioning as molecular organizers of the cartilaginous extracellular matrix.

Articular cartilage is composed of several morphologically distinct components that extend from the articulating surface (adjacent to the joint space) to the subchondral bone. These cartilage layers, also known as zones, are involved in the formation of an articulating surface and the compression-resistance core of the tissue as well as its attachment to the subjacent bone (**Table 1**). Articular cartilage exhibits a gradation in matrix composition, collagen organization, and chondrocyte shape and aggregation from the articulating surface through to the underlying calcified cartilage, which varies with the process of cartilage maturation.

ARTICULAR-EPIPHYSEAL CARTILAGE (IMMATURE)

At birth, the immature articular cartilage is thick and vascular, occupying the majority of the epiphysis. With growth and development, the immature

Table 1
Summary of the main features of immature and mature cartilage

	Structure/ Macromolecules	Immature Cartilage (Children)	Mature Cartilage (Adult)
Articular cartilage	Extracellular matrix synthesis vs degradation	Synthesis outweighs degradation	Synthesis balanced by controlled matrix degradation
	Cartilage thickness	Thick cartilage that decreases with maturation	Relatively thin articular cartilage
	Cartilage morphology	4 distinct zones: Zone of articular cartilage Zone of proliferation Zone of maturation Zone of calcification	3 distinct zones of uncalcified cartilage: Superficial zone Middle zone Deep zone
	Tidemark	Absent initially but develops as the cartilage matures	Well-demarcated lamina
	Calcified zone	Absent	Hypertrophied chondrocytes embedded in calcified matrix
	Vascularity	Present but decreases with cartilage maturation	Avascular
Growth plate	Morphology	4 distinct zones: Zone of resting Zone of proliferation Zone of maturation Zone of calcification	Replaced by the primary tensile bone trabecula

cartilage forms a cap over the articulating ends of the epiphyses with the structural features of articular cartilage adjacent to the bursa (joint space) and epiphyseal cartilage adjacent to the subchondral bone of the epiphyses. The cartilaginous cap persists into adult life, whereas its epiphyseal component is lost.

The immature articular-epiphyseal cartilage show 4 morphologically distinct zones extending from the free surface to the subchondral bone, as follows (**Fig. 2**A, B): (a) the zone of articulating cartilage with characteristic features of a mature cartilage, and the subsequent zones typical of the epiphyseal cartilage consisting of: (b) the zone of proliferation with active chondrocytes undergoing mitosis, (c) the zone of maturation with hypertrophic chondrocytes that accumulate glycogen and lipid and secretes alkaline phosphatase to the surrounding extracellular matrix, and (d) the zone of calcification with necrotic chondrocytes and an extracellular matrix rich in insoluble salts with traces of bone trabeculae and vascular infiltration.

In children up to the time of growth cessation, the epiphyseal cartilage or growth plate is located between the epiphysis and metaphysis. The growth plate enables bone to grow to its adult length and then is obliterated once the adult bone length is attained. Frequently, toward the end stage of bone growth (adolescent children/young adult) the epiphyseal component of the articular cartilage is still present, whereas the growth-plate cartilage disappears. The same principle applies for all mammals (see **Table 1**). The growth plate consists of 4 merging zones (**Figs. 2**C, D; **3**), namely: (a) the zone of resting cartilage, which contains the inactive (resting) chondrocytes and functions to anchor the remaining growth plate to the epiphysis; (b) the zone of proliferation with cells actively undergoing mitosis, hence providing a continuing supply of new chondrocytes; (c) the zone of hypertrophy with enlarged cells containing glycogen and lipid; and (d) the zone of calcification that lies adjacent to the newly formed trabecular of the subchondral bone and characterized by necrotic chondrocytes embedded within calcified extracellular matrix.

ARTICULAR CARTILAGE (MATURE)

Adult articular cartilage is divided into 4 distinct zones: (a) the superficial zone, composed of thin

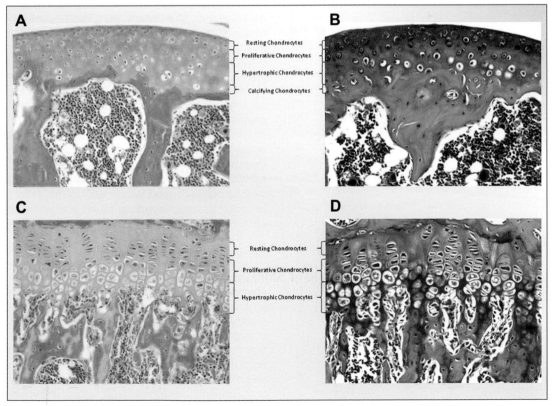

Fig. 2. Articular-epiphyseal cartilage (*A, B*) and the growth plate (*C, D*) of a 12-week-old wild-type mouse. Histologic sections were stained with hematoxylin and eosin (H&E; *A, C*) and with Toluidine Blue (*B, D*). The Toluidine Blue stain shows the following structures, which are observed during endochondral ossification: cartilage (*magenta*), calcified cartilage (*purple*), and bone (*blue*) (original magnification ×40).

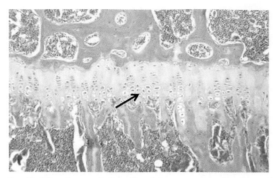

Fig. 3. Histology of the distal femur growth plate of a 12-week-old wild-type mouse, showing the various morphologic zones of differentiated chondrocytes. The arrow is indicating hypertrophic chondrocytes prior to the process of endochondral ossification. The growth plate enables bone to grow to its adult length through the process of endochondral ossification (H&E, original magnification ×10).

collagen fibrils arranged parallel to the surface, and associated with a high concentration of decorin and a low concentration of aggrecan[10]; (b) the middle (transitional) zone, with thick collagen fibrils arranged as gothic arches; (c) the deep (radial) zone, in which the collagen bundles are thickest and are arranged in a radial fashion; and (d) the calcified cartilage zone, located between the tidemark (the interface between the uncalcified cartilage and the calcified cartilage) and the subchondral bone. The structural integrity between the more compliant articular cartilage and the rigid calcified cartilage beneath is achieved by a continuity of collagen fibers across the interface.[11] The tidemark and the calcified cartilage serve as an interface between articular cartilage and underlying subchondral bone (**Fig. 4**); this functions as a physical barrier for nutrient diffusion and vascularization. This interface also serves as a zone of decreased compliance, thereby facilitating the

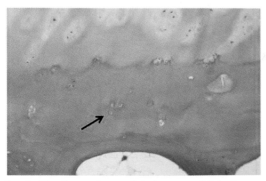

Fig. 4. Histology of an adult human tibial plateau, showing the calcified cartilage and tidemark. The arrow shows chondrocytes embedded in the calcified matrix. (H&E, original magnification ×20).

pressurization and physiologic loading of articular cartilage.[12] The tidemark is typically absent in immature cartilage.

CHONDROGENESIS

Articular cartilage is a highly specialized connective tissue derived from the mesenchymal lineage. The process of chondrogenesis consists of a highly orchestrated series of events that is initiated through the precursor mesenchymal cell stimulation, followed by highly organized cellular condensation and differentiation of mesenchymal cells to chondrocytes along with secretion of extracellular matrix (**Fig. 5**). During skeletal development, chondrogenesis is a crucial process that determines the shape and size of definitive bones in vertebrates, and results in the formation of a cartilage template (also known as the cartilage model).[13–15] Chondrogenesis is then followed by a process called endochondral ossification, which includes programmed cell death and the gradual replacement of most of the cartilage model by bone formation.

Precursor Mesenchymal Cells

Mesenchymal stem cells are multipotent stem cells that can differentiate into a variety of multiple lineages and specialized cell types, including: chondrocytes, osteoblasts (bone-forming cells), adipocytes (fat cells), and myocytes (muscle cells), based on specific genetic and molecular stimulations both in vivo and in vitro.[16–18] At the initiation of limb development, undifferentiated mesenchymal cells in the lateral plate mesoderm receive proliferation signals from the apical ectodermal ridge. Before condensation, the prechondrocytic mesenchymal stem cells produce extracellular matrix rich in hyaluronan and collagen type I, as well as collagen type IIA containing the exon 2–encoded amino-propeptide found in noncartilage collagens.[19]

Mesenchymal Condensation

The aggregation of chondroprogenitor mesenchymal cells into precartilage condensations (**Fig. 6**), first described by Fell, represents an early event in chondrogenesis.[20,21] The mesenchymal condensation involves an active cellular movement that causes an increase in mesenchymal cell aggregation in close apposition with one another and migration into the core of the embryonic limb bud, resulting in an increase in cells per unit volume without an increase in cell proliferation.[15,22,23] This event favors an increase in cell-cell contacts, and interaction through cell-cell adhesion molecules and gap junctions. In parallel, cells peripheral to

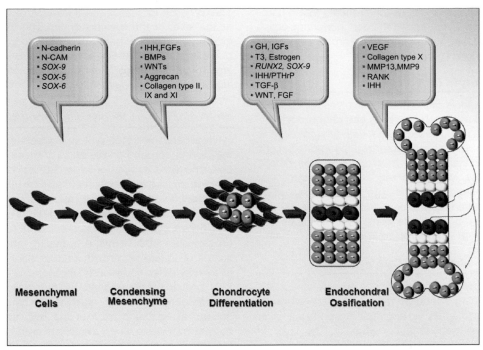

Fig. 5. Schematic diagram showing the various stages of chondrogenesis and endochondral ossification along with the key factors (proteins/genes) involved at each stage. The process of chondrogenesis is initiated with the stimulation of mesenchymal stem cells to differentiate to prechondrocytic cells, which migrate and condense to form cartilage template for the formation of long bones. Then the cells differentiate into chondrocytes and start to proliferate. Finally, the process of endochondral ossification starts with vascular penetration, forming the primary center of ossification followed by the secondary center of ossification. BMP, bone morphogenetic protein; FGF, fibroblast growth factor; GH, growth hormone; IGF, insulin-like growth factor; IHH, Indian hedgehog homologue; MMP, matrix metalloproteinase; N-CAM, neural cell adhesion molecule; PTHrP, parathyroid hormone–related peptide; RANK, receptor activator of nuclear factor κB; TGF, transforming growth factor; VEGF, vascular endothelial growth factor.

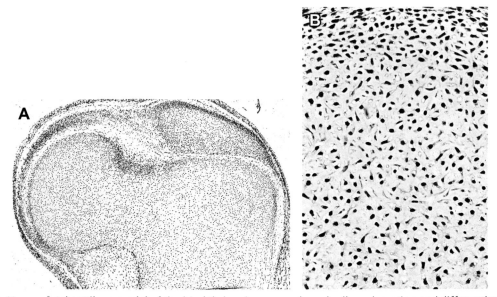

Fig. 6. Human fetal cartilage model of the hip (*A*) showing mesenchymal cell condensation and differentiation to prechondrocytic cells (*B*). (Original magnification, A × 2 and B × 40).

the condensation region differentiate into a fibro-blastic cell layer, termed the perichondrium, which in turn differentiates into bone-producing osteo-blasts, forming the periosteum.[24]

Chondrocyte Differentiation

Chondrogenic differentiation involves the specialization of mesenchymal cells into chondrocytes.[25] Each stage of mesenchymal cell differentiation to chondrocytes is characterized by modifications in cell proliferation, morphology, and biosynthetic activity as well as secretion of the extracellular matrix macromolecules. The matrix produced by differentiated chondrocytes is essential for the formation of the future bone as it maintains and regulates the chondrocyte phenotype.

Growth of Articular Cartilage

The embryonic chondroblast (early-stage, actively synthesizing chondrocyte) secretes the extracellular matrix at its vicinity, forming a fibrous layer known as perichondrium (**Fig. 7**). The layer of chondroblasts underneath the fibrous perichondrium secretes the cartilaginous matrix and embeds the chondroblasts, which are then termed chondrocytes. Eventually a cartilage template is formed, which persists during fetal life (see **Fig. 6**).

The growth of cartilage occurs by 2 independent mechanisms, both of which can occur simultaneously, namely the appositional growth and the interstitial growth. The appositional growth occurs at the chondrogenic level of the perichondrium where new layers of the extracellular matrix are formed on the surface of the existing cartilage.

This process increases the thickness of cartilage at the level of the perichondrium. The interstitial growth, on the other hand, involves mitotic division of the existing chondrocytes and secretion of cartilage matrix by the daughter chondrocytes, resulting in the growth of the matrix surrounding the cells.

Molecular Factors Involved in Chondrogenesis

Several genes and their protein expression pattern the distribution and proliferation of mesenchymal condensations at sites of future skeletal elements (see **Fig. 5**). The molecular mechanisms underlying this complex process have been studied extensively.[26,27] Several transcription factors such as Sox genes and Runx genes are crucial for chondrogenesis. Also, several signaling molecules including fibroblast growth factors (FGFs, such as FGF8), Indian hedgehog (IHH), bone morphogenetic protein (BMP), and the Wnt pathway regulate chondrogenesis through highly coordinated interactions along the 3 axes of the limb to ensure correct patterning along the dorsoventral and anteroposterior axes.[26,27] Expression of genes encoding these signaling molecules are mutually regulated, and the proper limb development consists of the cooperative integration of these 3 axes.[15]

Sox9 is a transcription factor with a high-mobility group DNA-binding domain that is expressed in all osteo-chondroprogenitors and plays an essential role in chondrogenesis.[28,29] Sox9 regulates the differentiation pathways of chondrocytes and osteoblasts, and also activates chondrocyte-specific marker genes, such as *Col2α1*, *Col11α2*, and

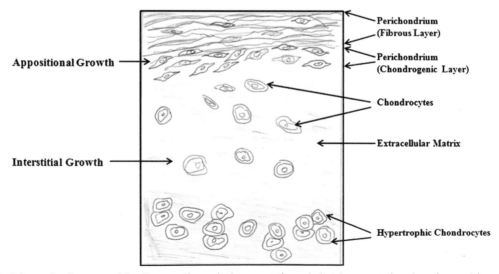

Fig. 7. Schematic diagram of hyaline cartilage during growth and development showing the perichondrium, extracellular matrix, and chondrocytes. (*Courtesy of* Dr Harpal K. Gahunia).

aggrecan.[30–32] Sox9 is expressed in all chondro-progenitors and chondrocytes except hypertrophic chondrocytes.[33] Inactivation of Sox9 during or after mesenchymal condensations causes severe chondrodysplasia, resulting in an almost complete absence of cartilage in the endochondral skeleton.[34] Furthermore, a heterozygous mutation in the Sox9 gene has been shown to result in campomelic dysplasia, which is characterized by a general hypoplasia of the endochondral bones.[35,36]

The family of Runx, a transcription factor that regulates chondrocyte differentiation, shares a highly homologous DNA-binding domain. The expression of these genes at precise times during skeletal development and chondrocyte differentiation is important, with each gene playing a distinct role in the differentiation of chondrocytes.[37–39] Specifically, Runx2 and Runx3 are important regulators of chondrocyte hypertrophy, whereas Runx1 are most likely required only in the very early stages of chondrocyte differentiation.[40] Overexpression of Runx1, Runx2, or Runx3 in nonhypertrophic chondrocytes leads to skeletal abnormalities.

FGFs play important roles in the control of embryonic and postnatal skeletal development by activating signaling through FGF receptors (FGFRs). A complex pattern of spatial regulation of FGFs and FGFRs in the different zones of the growth plate has been documented.[41] FGFs can substitute for the apical ridge and promote limb bud outgrowth and patterning.[42] Cross-talk between the FGFR pathway and other signaling cascades controls mesenchymal cell differentiation. Cellular differentiation of mesenchymal cells into subtypes with different FGFRs occurs in the presence of spatio-temporal variations of FGFs and transforming growth factor β (TGF-β).[43] FGF2, FGF4, and FGF6 have been used in vitro with TGF-β to increase the proliferation and induce the differentiation of mesenchymal cells to chondrocytes.[44] FGF and Wnt signals act together to synergistically promote proliferation; whereas, withdrawal of both signals results in cell-cycle withdrawal and chondrogenic differentiation.[45] Genetic analyses during mouse craniofacial skeletogenesis have shown that the interplay between Wnt and FGFR1 determines the fate and differentiation of mesenchymal cells. Mutations in FGFR constitutively activate FGFR signaling, causing chondrocytes and osteoblast dysfunctions that result in skeletal dysplasias.

In mammals, the TGF-β superfamily consists of about 30 structurally related proteins; these include 3 isoforms of TGF-β itself, 3 forms of activin, and more than 20 BMPs. TGF-β is critical for maintenance of synovial joints and is among the earliest signal in chondrogenic condensation. The initiation of condensation is associated with increased hyaluronidase activity and with the involvement of 2 cell adhesion molecules, N-cadherin[46] and neural cell adhesion molecule (N-CAM),[22] which are Ca^{2+}-dependent and Ca^{2+}-independent cell-cell adhesion molecules, respectively.[47] TGF-β stimulates the synthesis of fibronectin (which in turn regulates N-CAM) and the cell-surface adhesion protein N-cadherin.[48,49] Increased concentrations of TGF-β establish fibronectin-rich domains and cause the cells within these domains to be sorted out from the surrounding mesenchyme to form direct cell-cell adhesion, resulting in mesenchymal condensation.[22] Syndecan binds to fibronectin and downregulates N-CAM, thereby setting the condensation boundaries.[22] Disruption of TGF-β signaling stimulates chondrocytes to increase their biosynthetic organelles, enlarging the cell, and to secrete more structural matrix molecules, resulting in articular cartilage to hypertrophy. Loss of responsiveness to TGF-β promotes terminal differentiation of chondrocytes and alterations of the cartilage matrix.[50,51] N-cadherin and N-CAM disappear in differentiating chondrocytes and are detectable later only in perichondrial cells. The extracellular matrix molecules such as tenascins and thrombospondins, including cartilage oligomeric matrix protein (COMP), interact with the cell adhesion molecules to activate intracellular signaling pathways involving focal adhesion kinase and paxillin, to initiate the transition from chondroprogenitor cells to a fully committed chondrocyte.[15]

BMPs are members of the TGF-β superfamily that play an important role in the initiation of cartilage formation.[52] To date, almost 30 BMPs have been described and classified into several subgroups according to their structural similarities. Within the developing limb cartilage model, BMP-2, -4, and -7 have been detected in the perichondrium. Activation of the TGF-β pathway is necessary for subsequent induction of chondrogenesis by BMPs.[53] The interaction between Activin-TGF-β and BMP pathways promotes the expression of SOX9 along with a local decrease in cell proliferation.[54] Barna and Niswander[55] demonstrated that BMP signaling leads to compaction of mesenchymal cells, regulating the cell cohesion in condensations. Deletion of BMP-encoding genes such as BMP-2 and BMP-4 results in the loss of precartilaginous condensation,[56] whereas deletion of BMP receptors (BMPR) such as BMPR1a and BMPR1b leads to either the absence of most limb condensations or failure of mesenchymal cells to differentiate into chondrocytes.[57]

Following cellular condensation the cells start differentiating into chondrocytes, a process associated with expression of cartilage-specific genes. These genes include components of cartilage extracellular matrix genes, such as those encoding collagen type II α1 (Col2α1), collagen type IX, collagen type XI, aggrecan, COMP, and LINK protein (which stabilize the proteoglycan aggregate in ground substance of cartilage matrix).[13] Expression of these genes is regulated at the transcriptional level, spatially and temporally, so that they have different and dynamic expression patterns during chondrogenic differentiation. Cells undergoing chondrogenesis acquire a distinct spherical cell morphology and initiate expression of the transcription factors SOX9, SOX5, and SOX6, which regulate the genes encoding the cartilage matrix molecules, collagen type II and aggrecan.[58] Subsequently, the chondrocytes proliferate and secrete a cartilage-specific matrix within which the cells are encased to form the cartilage model. This matrix contains collagen type II,[59–63] collagen types IX and XI,[63–65] GLA protein,[66–68] aggrecan (large chondroitin sulfate–rich proteoglycan),[10,69–71] and LINK protein,[72] while the expression of collagen type I is turned off.

ENDOCHONDRAL OSSIFICATION

Endochondral ossification is a complex process by which the cartilaginous model formed during fetal life provides the template and contributes to the longitudinal growth of the long bones postnally.[50,73] This process occurs first at the center of the cartilaginous model and later at each end by a mixture of cells that establish the primary and secondary centers of ossification in the diaphysis and epiphysis, respectively.[73]

With continued growth of the cartilage model (through interstitial and appositional growth), the chondrocytes in its midsection hypertrophy, and with vascular penetration the hypertrophied chondrocytes begins to calcify, resulting in the formation of bone collar under the periosteum. When the calcified cartilage begins to break down, periosteal capillaries with osteogenic cells penetrate to establish the primary center of ossification in the diaphysis (mid-shaft of long bone). This process initiates the formation of the medullary cavity. Through a similar process the epiphyseal centers of ossification develop at the ends of the long bone postnatally.

Although the process of endochondral ossification begins during fetal life, the articular cartilage covering the ends of long bone emerges postnatally, and its maturation is completed by adulthood. Appearance of articular cartilage occurs at 2 weeks postnatally, when a small domain of secondary ossification occurs in the center of the epiphysis, separating the articular cartilage from the growth-plate cartilage.[74]

The epiphyseal cartilage component at the articular surface and growth plate plays an essential role in the development and growth of long bones.[75] At this stage, the deep zone of the newly formed articular cartilage is a growth plate–like tissue that contains a thin layer of enlarged chondrocytes expressing collagen type X (ColX), which is essential for formation of the calcified zone seen in adult articular cartilage. ColX assembly into a lattice-like network around hypertrophic chondrocytes is required for retaining or trapping the essential cartilage matrix components, including matrix vesicles and proteoglycans that promote initiation of normal mineralization. By 1 month of age, the secondary ossification center is expanded and the calcified zone starts to be formed.

In the growth plate, the zone of resting chondrocytes forms a template that attaches to the epiphyses, hence supporting the growth plate itself. The chondrocytes in this zone act as the reserve stem-like cells that replenish the pool of proliferative chondrocytes.[76] Some groups suggest that resting zone cartilage cells also contribute to endochondral bone formation by producing a growth plate–orienting factor (morphogen) that directs the alignment of the proliferative clones into columns parallel to the long axis of the bone, and by producing a morphogen that inhibits terminal differentiation of nearby proliferative zone chondrocytes, thus helping to organize the growth plate into distinct zones of proliferation and hypertrophy.[77]

Adjacent to the zone of resting chondrocytes is the zone of proliferation, where the chondrocytes replicate at a high rate and line up along the long axis of the bone. Following proliferation, chondrocytes pass through a transition stage in which they are known as prehypertrophic chondrocytes. Then, at the zone of hypertrophy, the chondrocytes increase in size by about 6- to 10 fold and secrete extracellular matrix that eventually becomes mineralized.[73] The area of hypertrophic cartilage is invaded by blood vessels, bone marrow cells, osteoclasts, macrophages, and osteoblasts, the last of which deposit bone on remnants of cartilage matrix.[78] At the zone of calcification, the hypertrophic chondrocytes undergo apoptosis shortly before the blood vessels invade the chondrocyte lacunae (**Figs. 8** and **9**).[79]

Molecular Factors Involved in Endochondral Ossification

The cells forming the cartilage model interzone are elongated in shape, are in direct contact with each other, and lose collagen type II expression while

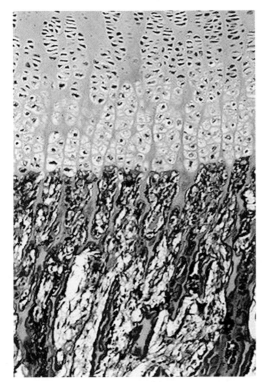

Fig. 8. Human epiphyseal cartilage showing the zone of proliferation, zone of maturation, zone of calcification, and new bone formation (H&E, original magnification ×40).

acquiring collagen type I immunoreactivity.[80] The 3-layered interzone has a dense intermediate cell layer and 2 outer cell layers, each facing the epiphyseal end of adjacent long-bone cartilage model.[81] Programmed cell death occurs within the interzone. The outer interzone layers participate in initial lengthening of long bone. However, cells within the intermediate high-density layer of the interzone are excluded from this process, and develop into the permanent layers of articular cartilage found in the mature joint.[82]

Chondrocytes in the zones of proliferation, hypertrophy, and calcification are essential regulators of skeletal development.[83,84] The regulation of endochondral ossification, which involves changes in chondrocyte behavior and is coordinated with the actions of blood vessels, osteoclasts, and osteoblasts, is subject to the influence of a plethora of extracellular factors, including TGF-β and the Wnt family of proteins, as well as components of the cartilage extracellular matrix. Wnt, TGF-β, and BMP protein family members are molecular regulators, and interactions of these 3 families have been extensively documented.[45,47,48,53] Understanding these interactions and their molecular targets is essential because chondrocytes in the epiphyseal cartilage simultaneously integrate these various complex signals.

Members of the TGF-β superfamily are secreted growth factors that regulate many aspects of

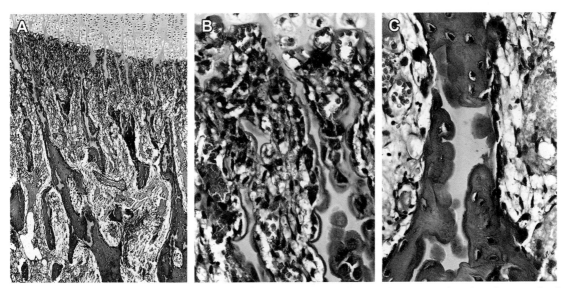

Fig. 9. (*A*) Human epiphyseal cartilage showing the zone of maturation with hypertrophic chondrocytes (*top*) and zone of calcification with necrotic chondrocytes and degraded cartilage matrix. (*B*) Zone of calcification showing calcification of the cartilage matrix and the replacement of the cartilaginous extracellular matrix by newly formed bone. (*C*) Osteoid tissue with osteoblasts on the surface and osteocytes embedded of newly formed bone matrix. Of note is the remnant of the cartilage matrix (*light pink stain at the center*) of the developing trabeculae (H&E, original magnification: A × 10, B and C × 100).

development, including cellular growth and differentiation. The cartilage interzone is an important signaling center, regulating growth through factors with chondrogenic activity such as growth differentiation factor 5 (GDF-5). Overexpression of GDF-5 during early skeletal development increases chondrocyte proliferation and increases the length of skeletal elements. Mutations in GDF-5 result in the autosomal recessive syndromes Hunter-Thompson and Grebe-type chondrodysplasias in humans.[85,86]

Transforming growth factor β

During skeletal development, TGF-β has unique functions and acts sequentially to modulate chondrocyte and osteoblast differentiation.[87] Specifically, TGF-β promotes chondrogenesis in cultures of undifferentiated multipotent mesenchymal cells, but inhibits hypertrophic differentiation of chondrocyte cultures and cultured long-bone rudiments of mice.[50]

TGF-βs maintain cartilage homeostasis by preventing inappropriate chondrocyte differentiation. TGF-β1, TGF-β2, and TGF-β3 cause arrest in the G1 phase of the cell cycle in many nontransformed cell types in vitro, and they also stimulate matrix production by mesenchymal cells.[87] TGF-βs signal through heteromeric type I and type II receptor serine/threonine. Transgenic mice with a defective TGF-β type II receptor develop progressive skeletal degeneration with replacement of the articular surfaces by bone and hypertrophic cartilage.[50] Noggin is a protein that in humans is encoded by the NOG gene. Noggin inhibits TGF-β transduction by binding to TGF-β family ligands and preventing them from binding to their corresponding receptors.[88]

Bone morphogenetic proteins

BMPs are multifunctional growth factors that play critical roles at various stages of skeletal development. BMPs were originally identified as proteins that ectopically stimulate cartilage and bone formation in vivo, but are now recognized as important regulators of growth, differentiation, and morphogenesis during embryology.[89] BMP-6 has been reported in prehypertrophic and hypertrophic chondrocytes, whereas BMP-7 was detected in chick sternal prehypertrophic and mouse metatarsal proliferating chondrocytes.[52]

BMPs act sequentially in regulating specific aspects of endochondral bone development. BMP signaling supports proliferation of chondrocytes in the growth plate. The cartilage interzone expresses both BMPs and their antagonists, such as Noggin, that are thought to interact with and modulate BMP activities. In mice lacking noggin, cartilage condensations are initiated normally but develop hyperplasia, with unaffected cartilage maturation. Excess BMP activity in the absence of noggin antagonism increased the recruitment of cells into cartilage, expanding the cartilage at the expense of other tissues, resulting in oversized growth plates and failure to initiate joint formation.[88] However, the effects of BMP signaling on chondrocyte hypertrophy is poorly understood. More than one subgroup of BMPs regulate to signal the stimulation of chondrocyte maturation, to increase IHH expression independent of maturational effects and to partially overcome the inhibitory effects of parathyroid hormone–related peptide (PTHrP) on maturation.[90–94]

Wnt family

The Wnt family of proteins consists of at least 22 cysteine-rich, secreted glyco/proteins (39- to 46-kDa) that drive developmentally important signaling pathways contributing to cell fate determination, spatial-temporal patterning, and cell motility. The Wnt signaling pathway is best known for its roles in embryogenesis and cancer. Wnt proteins play an important role in development and maintenance of many organs and tissues, including bone and cartilage.[95,96] In the skeletal system, Wnt-signaling functions are complex. During the development of vertebrate long bone, Wnt and FGF signals interact to coordinate growth of the multipotent progenitor cells with their simultaneous segregation into a chondrogenic lineage (located in the center of the cartilage model), and connective tissue lineage at the periphery of the limb bud.[45] Wnt and FGF signals act synergistically to promote proliferation while maintaining the cells in an undifferentiated, multipotent state. However, they also act independently to determine the specification of cell lineage. Withdrawal of both signals results in chondrogenic differentiation, whereas continued exposure to Wnt maintains proliferation and respecifies the cells toward the lineages of soft connective tissue.

Overexpression of Wnt4 in the developing chick limb promotes chondrocyte hypertrophy, resulting in shortened skeletal elements with an expanded bone collar.[97] Wnt9α (formerly known as Wnt14), expressed in the developing joint interzone, has been implicated in the initial steps of synovial joint formation.[98] The expression of Wnt9a and Wnt4 precedes or coincides with the downregulation of collagen type II (Col2α1) and SOX9. The downregulation of these chondrogenic markers during joint formation suggested that an essential step in joint formation is to block the further differentiation of these cells into chondrocytes.[99]

Several studies have shown that Wnt/β-catenin signaling is active during endochondral bone formation and stimulates chondrocyte maturation.[99–101] Wnt4 and β-catenin, expressed in the joint interzone and articular cartilage, may accelerate chondrocyte hypertrophy. The Wnt/β-catenin pathway seems to be important in maintaining joint identity by actively suppressing the chondrogenic potential in precursor cells. Wnt4 has been thought to directly promote terminal differentiation, and its role in the joint may be distinct. Wnt/β-catenin signaling inhibits chondrogenesis in the developing skeleton.[101] Subsequently, β-catenin signaling is reestablished in the growth plate, where numerous Wnts are expressed once cartilage has formed and the skeletal elements have developed.[102] Wnt/β-catenin signaling also facilitates the formation of hypertrophic chondrocytes through the induction of the transcription factor *RUNX2*.[103] Cell culture and chick limb-bud models suggest that Wnt/β-catenin signaling stimulates chondrocyte maturation. Overexpression of Wnts 4, 8, and 9, β-catenin, and *LEF*-1 induce collagen type X, alkaline phosphatase, and other genes associated with chondrocyte hypertrophy.

Noncanonical Wnt signaling acts independently of β-catenin, and increases intracellular calcium concentrations or controls cell polarity by activation of Rho guanosine triphosphatases. The Wnt/Ca^{2+} pathway regulates cell movements in the early stage of development.[104] Wnt5a and Wnt11 regulate cartilage-specific extracellular matrix molecule synthesis through the noncanonical pathway.[105]

CARTILAGE MATRIX MODELING DURING ENDOCHONDRAL OSSIFICATION

The key features of endochondral ossification involve cartilage extracellular matrix degradation and mineralization, which is a tightly regulated mechanism whereby several molecules play variable roles in a well-orchestrated manner. A triad of factors is essential for a proper cartilage matrix modeling, a process that encompasses hypertrophic chondrocyte differentiation, vascular invasion, and proteolytic activity. The axis "chondrocyte hypertrophy–matrix mineralization" involves both secreting factors (such as vascular endothelial growth factor [VEGF] and matrix metalloproteinases [MMPs]) and key signaling members (such as Wnt/β-catenin and PTHrP-IHH).

The cascade of events is initiated when the extracellular matrix produced by the most advanced hypertrophic chondrocytes becomes mineralized, during which the terminal hypertrophic chondrocytes undergo apoptosis and are replaced by the bone cells.[106] Vascular invasion is facilitated by VEGF, establishing a strong gradient of angiogenic factors. This process is accompanied by changes in the extracellular matrix synthesis, such as upregulation of collagen type X and MMP-13 in hypertrophic chondrocytes.

In addition to their contribution to bone growth, hypertrophic chondrocytes coordinate multiple aspects of endochondral ossification through their secreted products.[107] The extracellular matrix deposited by hypertrophic chondrocytes serves as a template for subsequent bone formation, and these cells also secrete soluble proteins, including VEGF, IHH, and receptor activator of nuclear factor κB (RANK) ligand, which control the activities of other cell lineages (endothelial cells, osteoblasts, and osteoclasts) involved in endochondral ossification.[78] All these factors synergistically degrade the extracellular matrix gradually and allow the further invasion of blood vessels and osteoclast and osteoblast precursors, which in turn are the key participants in laying down bone tissue on the cartilage matrix template. In mice lacking VEGF expression by hypertrophic chondrocytes, both vascular invasion and mineralization are delayed.[108]

Chondrocyte hypertrophy, an essential step during endochondral bone formation, is tightly controlled during normal skeletal development by cell-cell signaling and transcription factors.[109,110] This process is initiated when the most central proliferating chondrocytes within the cartilage model exit the cell cycle and differentiate to hypertrophy. Hypertrophic chondrocytes increase 20-fold in cell size and cellular fluid volume.

IHH, an essential protein for endochondral ossification that synchronizes skeletal angiogenesis with perichondral maturation, is expressed in prehypertrophic chondrocytes as they enter the hypertrophic phase. During this phase, IHH begins to downregulate the expression of collagen type II and initiates expression of the hypertrophic chondrocyte markers collagen type X and alkaline phosphatase.[13] Hypertrophic chondrocytes mineralize their surrounding matrix and eventually undergo apoptosis while the area of hypertrophic cartilage is invaded by blood vessels, along with osteoclast and osteoblast precursor cells. Collectively these cells degrade, leaving a mineralized cartilage extracellular matrix template on which osteoblasts adhere. The osteoblasts then secrete the new bone matrix (osteoid) and regulate its calcification to bone tissue, forming a primary ossification center. The cartilage segments that remain on either side of the primary ossified region are termed the growth plates, and are responsible for the longitudinal growth of long bones.[8] The proper regulation of chondrocyte hypertrophy is also necessary for maintaining the cartilage lining synovial joint surfaces, as abnormal chondrocyte hypertrophy in articular cartilage is associated with osteoarthritis.[111]

TGF-β/BMP Signaling and Chondrocyte Hypertrophy

TGF-βs and their receptors are expressed during the development of the skeleton, and are known to regulate chondrocyte proliferation and differentiation.[112,113] TGF-β also plays a role as a regulator of chondrocyte maturation, maintaining cartilage homeostasis by preventing inappropriate chondrocyte differentiation. Loss of responsiveness to TGF-β results in abnormal terminal chondrocyte maturation with increased collagen type X–expressing hypertrophic chondrocytes, accompanied by dysfunctional matrix production. This view is consistent with the first observations showing that TGF-β prevents hypertrophic differentiation in chondrocytes grown in suspension and pellet cultures as well as in long-bone rudiment organ cultures.[114–116]

Smads are the intracellular mediators of TGF-β signaling. While Smad3 transduces TGF-β signals, Smad7 inhibits both TGF-β and BMP signaling.[117] Iwai and colleagues[117] found that Smad7 overexpression in conditional transgenic mice exerts specific functions at multiple stages of chondrocyte differentiation, decreasing proliferation and inhibiting maturation toward hypertrophy.

Wnt/β-Catenin Signaling in Cartilage Differentiation

Signaling by the Wnt family of secreted glycoproteins via the transcriptional coactivator β-catenin is one of the fundamental mechanisms that direct cell proliferation and determine cell fate during embryonic development and tissue homeostasis. Among the constituents of the β-catenin degradation complex, Axin is of particular interest. Axin1 and Axin2 have been shown to inhibit Wnt/β-catenin signaling and stimulate TGF-β signaling. Conversely, suppression of Axin1 and Axin2 enhances Wnt/β-catenin and reduces TGF-β signaling, resulting in an acceleration of chondrocyte maturation.[100]

The Wnt/β-catenin pathway is of key importance in articular cartilage homeostasis, whereby it regulates chondrocyte phenotype and maturation and performs a critical function for growth plate organization and endochondral ossification. β-Catenin signaling is required for proper cellular differentiation from cartilage to bone cells. Overexpression of Wnt14 is associated with chondrocyte hypertrophy, cartilage maturation, and endochondral bone formation.[118] Using transgenic mice expressing a fusion mutant protein β-catenin and

Lef, Tamamura and colleagues[119] showed that the growth plates were totally disorganized by lacking mature chondrocytes expressing IHH and collagen type X, and failing to undergo endochondral ossification. This observation was confirmed in cultured chondrocytes, where activation of β-catenin was associated with chondrocyte hypertrophy, matrix mineralization, and expression of terminal markers such as MMP-13 and VEGF.

Gaur and colleagues[120] investigated the role of canonical Wnt signaling in a mouse model in which the Wnt antagonist secreted Frizzled-related protein 1 (sFRP1) was nonfunctional. These investigators found shortened height of the growth plate and increased calcification of the hypertrophic zone in the sfrp1$^{-/-}$ mouse, indicating accelerated endochondral ossification. Wnt/β-catenin signaling is a contributing mechanism for increased chondrocyte hypertrophy and cartilage differentiation.[120] Wnt signaling may increase bone mass by keeping the osteoblasts in the proliferation phase.[121]

Overexpression of β-catenin in chondrocytes strongly stimulates the expression of matrix degradation enzymes.[122–126] Chen and colleagues[127] showed that conditional chondrocyte-specific deletion of β-catenin in adult mice leads to a rapid and profound degradation of cartilage. Moreover, inhibition of β-catenin signaling in articular chondrocytes in a transgenic mouse causes increased cell apoptosis and articular cartilage destruction.[128] Conversely, antagonists of Wnt, particularly FRZB-1, have a role in chondrocyte formation, suggesting that a balance between Wnt activators and antagonists is important for proper cartilage formation.[129]

Several extracellular proteins modulate the activity of the Wnt/β-catenin signaling pathway, including the Dickkopf family of proteins (Dkk-1, -2, -3, and -4), the sFRP, the Wnt-modulator in surface ectoderm protein, and the SOST gene product, sclerostin.[129,130]

Dickkopf Proteins

Dkk proteins are secreted glycoproteins that inhibit Wnt/β-catenin signaling. Mice overexpressing Dkk1 in osteoblasts develop osteopenia through reduced osteoblast number and bone formation, whereas Dkk2$^{-/-}$ mice are osteopenic, with increased osteoid and impaired mineralization. These mice showed enhanced osteoclastic activity with the upregulation of RANK ligand expression, indicating that Dkk2 affects both bone formation and bone resorption.[131]

Sclerostin

Sclerostin is a protein product of the SOST gene and is produced by the osteocytes. Sclerostin regulates the Wnt by inhibiting Wnt/β-catenin signaling, Mutations in this gene in humans have been shown to cause the disease of increased bone mass known as sclerosteosis. Targeting and overexpression of the *SOST* gene in mice lead to an increase and a reduction, respectively, in bone mass with altered bone formation.[130]

Matrix Metalloproteinases During Chondrocyte Hypertrophy

Several MMPs, a family of proteases, are expressed during endochondral ossification, including collagenases (MMP-1 and MMP-13), gelatinases (MMP-2 and MMP-9), stromelysins (MMP-3 and MMP-10), and an MT1-MMP. These proteases are able to cleave a variety of substrates including cartilage matrix proteins and cell surface proteins. Within the growth plate, MMP-13, which degrades both fibrillar collagen and aggrecan, is the major collagenase and is selectively expressed by hypertrophic chondrocytes.[132] MMP-13 transcription is controlled by *RUNX2*, both important participants in the axis "chondrocyte hypertrophy–matrix mineralization."[133] MMP-9, in contrast to MMP-13, does not cleave native fibrillar collagens, but does cleave denatured collagens and aggrecan.[132] MMP-9 is highly expressed in monocytes, preosteoclasts, and osteoclasts, and is concentrated at sites of cartilage resorption, where vascular invasion occurs.

SUMMARY

Chondrocytes synthesize and secrete the major macromolecular components of cartilage matrix and they can also degrade the matrix by releasing degradative enzymes such as collagenase and other metalloproteinases including stromelysin. During growth and development of immature cartilage, matrix synthesis outweighs the degradation. As a result, the ratio of extracellular matrix to chondrocytes in articular cartilage rises during growth to reach the mature adult level of about 20:1. In adults, matrix synthesis is finely balanced by controlled matrix degradation. In most growing individuals, the complex pattern of cartilage growth regulated by cascades of signaling molecules works seamlessly and without fail. However, disruption to the normal balance of synthesis and degradation can lead to variation in the intrinsic characteristics of cartilage matrix. Depending on the extent of the disorder, this can lead to a gradual degeneration of the extracellular matrix that is responsible for the genesis of clinically recognizable developmental cartilage diseases.

Advances in understanding of the age-related morphologic, biochemical, and biomechanical changes in articular cartilage (including growth plate) and their effects on joint homeostasis, the natural healing process after cartilage acute or chronic injury, and improved diagnostic standards for cartilage lesion evaluations makes the ultimate goal of cartilage repair a possibility. Furthermore, advances in tissue engineering as well as in treatment and surgical strategies have enhanced the limited healing potential of articular cartilage and the regeneration of repair tissue in chondral and osteochondral lesions. This article reviews developments in basic science and clinical research so as to provide a better understanding of the key molecular and genetic participants during the growth and development of articular cartilage. This knowledge is the basis for strategies currently being used to design emerging technologies for the treatment of articular cartilage defects and in cartilage-related diseases.

REFERENCES

1. Kuettner KE, Aydelotte MB, Thonar EJ. Articular cartilage matrix and structure: a minireview. J Rheumatol Suppl 1991;27:46–8.
2. Ghadially FN. Fine structure of the joint. In: Sokoloff L, editor. The joints and synovial fluid. New York: Academic Press; 1978. p. 105–76.
3. Ogata K, Whiteside LA. Barrier to material transfer at the bone-cartilage interface: measurement with hydrogen gas in vivo. Clin Orthop Relat Res 1979;145:273–6.
4. Visco DM, Van Sickle DC, Hill MA, et al. The vascular supply of the chondro-epiphyses of the elbow joint in young swine. J Anat 1989;163:215–29.
5. Clark JM. The structure of vascular channels in the subchondral plate. J Anat 1990;171:105–15.
6. Jackson A, Gu W. Transport properties of cartilaginous tissues. Curr Rheumatol Rev 2009;5:40.
7. Mow VC, Ratcliffe A, Poole AR. Cartilage and diarthrodial joints as paradigms for hierarchical materials and structures. Biomaterials 1992;13:67–97.
8. Woods A, Wang G, Beier F. Regulation of chondrocyte differentiation by the actin cytoskeleton and adhesive interactions. J Cell Physiol 2007;213:1–8.
9. Goldring MB, Marcu KB. Cartilage homeostasis in health and rheumatic diseases. Arthritis Res Ther 2009;11:224.
10. Mallein-Gerin F, Kosher RA, Upholt WB, et al. Temporal and spatial analysis of cartilage proteoglycan core protein gene expression during limb development by in situ hybridization. Dev Biol 1988;126:337–45.
11. Broom ND, Poole CA. A functional-morphological study of the tidemark region of articular cartilage maintained in a non-viable physiological condition. J Anat 1982;135:65–82.

12. Redler I, Mow VC, Zimny ML, et al. The ultrastructure and biomechanical significance of the tidemark of articular cartilage. Clin Orthop Relat Res 1975;(112):357–62.

13. Goldring MB, Tsuchimochi K, Ijiri K. The control of chondrogenesis. J Cell Biochem 2006;97: 33–44.

14. de Crombrugghe B, Lefebvre V, Behringer RR, et al. Transcriptional mechanisms of chondrocyte differentiation. Matrix Biol 2000;19:389–94.

15. DeLise AM, Fischer L, Tuan RS. Cellular interactions and signaling in cartilage development. Osteoarthritis Cartilage 2000;8:309–34.

16. Teven CM, Liu X, Hu N, et al. Epigenetic regulation of mesenchymal stem cells: a focus on osteogenic and adipogenic differentiation. Stem Cells Int 2011; 2011:201371.

17. Viero Nora CC, Camassola M, Bellagamba B, et al. Molecular analysis of the differentiation potential of murine mesenchymal stem cells from tissues of endodermal or mesodermal origin. Stem Cells Dev 2011. [Epub ahead of print].

18. da Silva Meirelles L, Chagastelles PC, Nardi NB. Mesenchymal stem cells reside in virtually all postnatal organs and tissues. J Cell Sci 2006;119: 2204–13.

19. Sandell LJ, Nalin AM, Reife RA. Alternative splice form of type II procollagen mRNA (IIA) is predominant in skeletal precursors and non-cartilaginous tissues during early mouse development. Dev Dyn 1994;199:129–40.

20. Fell HB. The histogenesis of cartilage and bone in the long bones of the embryonic fowl. J Morphol Physiol 1925;40:417–59.

21. Thorogood PV, Hinchliffe JR. An analysis of the condensation process during chondrogenesis in the embryonic chick hind limb. J Embryol Exp Morphol 1975;33:581–606.

22. Hall BK, Miyake T. All for one and one for all: condensations and the initiation of skeletal development. Bioessays 2000;22:138–47.

23. Janners MY, Searls RL. Changes in rate of cellular proliferation during the differentiation of cartilage and muscle in the mesenchyme of the embryonic chick wing. Dev Biol 1970;23:136–65.

24. Erlebacher A, Filvaroff EH, Gitelman SE, et al. Toward a molecular understanding of skeletal development. Cell 1995;80:371–8.

25. Olsen BR, Reginato AM, Wang W. Bone development. Annu Rev Cell Dev Biol 2000;16:191–220.

26. Tickle C. Molecular basis of vertebrate limb patterning. Am J Med Genet 2002;112:250–5.

27. Shimizu H, Yokoyama S, Asahara H. Growth and differentiation of the developing limb bud from the perspective of chondrogenesis. Dev Growth Differ 2007;49:449–54.

28. Akiyama H, Kim JE, Nakashima K, et al. Osteochondroprogenitor cells are derived from Sox9 expressing precursors. Proc Natl Acad Sci U S A 2005;102:14665–70.

29. Ng LJ, Wheatley S, Muscat GE, et al. SOX9 binds DNA, activates transcription, and coexpresses with type II collagen during chondrogenesis in the mouse. Dev Biol 1997;183:108–21.

30. Lefebvre V, Huang W, Harley VR, et al. SOX9 is a potent activator of the chondrocyte-specific enhancer of the pro alpha1(II) collagen gene. Mol Cell Biol 1997;17:2336–46.

31. Sekiya I, Tsuji K, Koopman P, et al. SOX9 enhances aggrecan gene promoter/enhancer activity and is up-regulated by retinoic acid in a cartilage-derived cell line, TC6. J Biol Chem 2000;275:10738–44.

32. Bridgewater LC, Lefebvre V, de Crombrugghe B. Chondrocyte-specific enhancer elements in the Col11a2 gene resemble the Col2a1 tissue-specific enhancer. J Biol Chem 1998;273:14998–5006.

33. Zhao Q, Eberspaecher H, Lefebvre V, et al. Parallel expression of Sox9 and Col2a1 in cells undergoing chondrogenesis. Dev Dyn 1997;209:377–86.

34. Akiyama H, Chaboissier MC, Martin JF, et al. The transcription factor Sox9 has essential roles in successive steps of the chondrocyte differentiation pathway and is required for expression of Sox5 and Sox6. Genes Dev 2002;16:2813–28.

35. Foster JW, Dominguez-Steglich MA, Guioli S, et al. Campomelic dysplasia and autosomal sex reversal caused by mutations in an SRY-related gene. Nature 1994;372:525–30.

36. Wagner T, Wirth J, Meyer J, et al. Autosomal sex reversal and campomelic dysplasia are caused by mutations in and around the SRY-related gene SOX9. Cell 1994;79:1111–20.

37. Sato S, Kimura A, Ozdemir J, et al. The distinct role of the Runx proteins in chondrocyte differentiation and intervertebral disc degeneration: findings in murine models and in human disease. Arthritis Rheum 2008;58:2764–75.

38. Stricker S, Fundele R, Vortkamp A, et al. Role of Runx genes in chondrocyte differentiation. Dev Bio 2002;245:95–108.

39. Yoshida CA, Yamamoto H, Fujita T, et al. Runx2 and Runx3 are essential for chondrocyte maturation, and Runx2 regulates limb growth through induction of Indian hedgehog. Genes Dev 2004; 18:952–63.

40. Wang Y, Belflower RM, Dong YF, et al. Runx1/ AML1/Cbfa2 mediates onset of mesenchymal cell differentiation toward chondrogenesis. J Bone Miner Res 2005;20:1624–36.

41. Lazarus JE, Hegde A, Andrade AC, et al. Fibroblast growth factor expression in the postnatal growth plate. Bone 2007;40:577–86.

42. Niswander L. Pattern formation: old models out on a limb. Nat Rev Genet 2003;4:133–43.

43. Hentschel HG, Glimm T, Glazier JA, et al. Dynamical mechanisms for skeletal pattern formation in the vertebrate limb. Proc Biol Sci 2004;271: 1713–22.

44. Miraoui H, Marie PJ. Fibroblast growth factor receptor signaling crosstalk in skeletogenesis. Sci Signal 2010;3:re9.

45. ten Berge D, Brugmann SA, Helms JA, et al. Wnt and FGF signals interact to coordinate growth with cell fate specification during limb development. Development 2008;135:3247–57.

46. Delise AM, Tuan RS. Analysis of N-cadherin function in limb mesenchymal chondrogenesis in vitro. Dev Dyn 2002;225:195–204.

47. Tuan RS. Cellular signaling in developmental chondrogenesis: N-cadherin, Wnts, and BMP-2. J Bone Joint Surg Am 2003;85(Suppl 2):137–41.

48. Leonard CM, Fuld HM, Frenz DA, et al. Role of transforming growth factor-beta in chondrogenic pattern formation in the embryonic limb: stimulation of mesenchymal condensation and fibronectin gene expression by exogenous TGF-beta and evidence for endogenous TGF-beta-like activity. Dev Biol 1991;145:99–109.

49. Tsonis PA, Del Rio-Tsonis K, Millan JL, et al. Expression of N-cadherin and alkaline phosphatase in chick limb bud mesenchymal cells: regulation by 1,25-dihydroxyvitamin D3 or TGF-beta 1. Exp Cell Res 1994;213:433–7.

50. Serra R, Johnson M, Filvaroff EH, et al. Expression of a truncated, kinase-defective TGF-beta type II receptor in mouse skeletal tissue promotes terminal chondrocyte differentiation and osteoarthritis. J Cell Biol 1997;139:541–52.

51. Yang X, Chen L, Xu X, et al. TGF-beta/Smad3 signals repress chondrocyte hypertrophic differentiation and are required for maintaining articular cartilage. J Cell Biol 2001;153:35–46.

52. van der Eerden BC, Karperien M, Wit JM. Systemic and local regulation of the growth plate. Endocr Rev 2003;24:782–801.

53. Karamboulas K, Dranse HJ, Underhill TM. Regulation of BMP-dependent chondrogenesis in early limb mesenchyme by TGFbeta signals. J Cell Sci 2010;123:2068–76.

54. Montero JA, Lorda-Diez CI, Ganan Y, et al. Activin/TGFbeta and BMP crosstalk determines digit chondrogenesis. Dev Biol 2008;321:343–56.

55. Barna M, Niswander L. Visualization of cartilage formation: insight into cellular properties of skeletal progenitors and chondrodysplasia syndromes. Dev Cell 2007;12:931–41.

56. Bandyopadhyay A, Tsuji K, Cox K, et al. Genetic analysis of the roles of BMP2, BMP4, and BMP7 in limb patterning and skeletogenesis. PLoS Genet 2006;2:e216.

57. Yoon BS, Ovchinnikov DA, Yoshii I, et al. Bmpr1a and Bmpr1b have overlapping functions and are essential for chondrogenesis in vivo. Proc Natl Acad Sci U S A 2005;102:5062–7.

58. Bi W, Deng JM, Zhang Z, et al. Sox9 is required for cartilage formation. Nat Genet 1999;22:85–9.

59. Kosher RA, Kulyk WM, Gay SW. Collagen gene expression during limb cartilage differentiation. J Cell Biol 1986;102:1151–6.

60. Kosher RA, Solursh M. Widespread distribution of type II collagen during embryonic chick development. Dev Biol 1989;131:558–66.

61. Kravis D, Upholt WB. Quantitation of type II procollagen mRNA levels during chick limb cartilage differentiation. Dev Biol 1985;108:164–72.

62. Nah HD, Rodgers BJ, Kulyk WM, et al. In situ hybridization analysis of the expression of the type II collagen gene in the developing chicken limb bud. Coll Relat Res 1988;8:277–94.

63. Swiderski RE, Solursh M. Localization of type II collagen, long form alpha 1(IX) collagen, and short form alpha 1(IX) collagen transcripts in the developing chick notochord and axial skeleton. Dev Dyn 1992;194:118–27.

64. Kulyk WM, Coelho CN, Kosher RA. Type IX collagen gene expression during limb cartilage differentiation. Matrix 1991;11:282–8.

65. Swiderski RE, Solursh M. Differential co-expression of long and short form type IX collagen transcripts during avian limb chondrogenesis in ovo. Development 1992;115:169–79.

66. Luo G, D'Souza R, Hogue D, et al. The matrix Gla protein gene is a marker of the chondrogenesis cell lineage during mouse development. J Bone Miner Res 1995;10:325–34.

67. Barone LM, Owen TA, Tassinari MS, et al. Developmental expression and hormonal regulation of the rat matrix Gla protein (MGP) gene in chondrogenesis and osteogenesis. J Cell Biochem 1991;46: 351–65.

68. Hale JE, Fraser JD, Price PA. The identification of matrix Gla protein in cartilage. J Biol Chem 1988; 263:5820–4.

69. Hascall VC, Oegema TR, Brown M. Isolation and characterization of proteoglycans from chick limb bud chondrocytes grown in vitro. J Biol Chem 1976;251:3511–9.

70. Palmoski MJ, Goetinck PF. Synthesis of proteochondroitin sulfate by normal, nanomelic, and 5-bromodeoxyuridine-treated chondrocytes in cell culture. Proc Natl Acad Sci U S A 1972;69: 3385–8.

71. Tsonis PA, Walker E. Cell populations synthesizing cartilage proteoglycan core protein in the early

chick limb bud. Biochem Biophys Res Commun 1991;174:688–95.

72. Stirpe NS, Goetinck PF. Gene regulation during cartilage differentiation: temporal and spatial expression of link protein and cartilage matrix protein in the developing limb. Development 1989; 07:23–33.

73. Mackie EJ, Ahmed YA, Tatarczuch L, et al. Endochondral ossification: how cartilage is converted into bone in the developing skeleton. Int J Biochem Cell Biol 2008;40:46–62.

74. Ortega N, Behonick DJ, Werb Z. Matrix remodeling during endochondral ossification. Trends Cell Biol 2004;4:86–93.

75. Archer CW, Francis-West P. The chondrocyte. Int J Biochem Cell Biol 2003;35:401–4.

76. Nilsson O, Marino R, De Luca F, et al. Endocrine regulation of the growth plate. Horm Res 2005;64: 157–65.

77. Abad V, Meyers JL, Weise M, et al. The role of the resting zone in growth plate chondrogenesis. Endocrinology 2002;143:1851–7.

78. Solomon LA, Berube NG, Beier F. Transcriptional regulators of chondrocyte hypertrophy. Birth Defects Res C Embryo Today 2008;84:123–30.

79. Farnum CE, Wilsman NJ. Cellular turnover at the chondro-osseous junction of growth plate cartilage: analysis by serial sections at the light microscopical level. J Orthop Res 1989;7:654–66.

80. Archer CW, Dowthwaite GP, Francis-West P. Development of synovial joints. Birth Defects Res C Embryo Today 2003;69:144–55.

81. Mitrovic D. Development of the diarthrodial joints in the rat embryo. Am J Anat 1978;151:475–85.

82. Ito MM, Kida MY. Morphological and biochemical re-evaluation of the process of cavitation in the rat knee joint: cellular and cell strata alterations in the interzone. J Anat 2000;197(Pt 4):659–79.

83. Haines RW. The development of joints. J Anat 1947;81:33–55.

84. Garciadiego-Cazares D, Rosales C, Katoh M, et al. Coordination of chondrocyte differentiation and joint formation by alpha5beta1 integrin in the developing appendicular skeleton. Development 2004; 131:4735–42.

85. Ploger F, Seemann P, Schmidt-von Kegler M, et al. Brachydactyly type A2 associated with a defect in proGDF5 processing. Hum Mol Genet 2008;17: 1222–33.

86. Francis-West PH, Abdelfattah A, Chen P, et al. Mechanisms of GDF-5 action during skeletal development. Development 1999;126:1305–15.

87. Moses HL, Serra R. Regulation of differentiation by TGF-beta. Curr Opin Genet Dev 1996;6: 581–6.

88. Brunet LJ, McMahon JA, McMahon AP, et al. Noggin, cartilage morphogenesis, and joint

89. Daans M, Lories RJ, Luyten FP. Dynamic activation of bone morphogenetic protein signaling in collagen-induced arthritis supports their role in joint homeostasis and disease. Arthritis Res Ther 2008; 10:R115.

90. Grimsrud CD, Romano PR, D'Souza M, et al. BMP-6 is an autocrine stimulator of chondrocyte differentiation. J Bone Miner Res 1999;14:475–82.

91. Minina E, Kreschel C, Naski MC, et al. Interaction of FGF, IHH/PTHLH, and BMP signaling integrates chondrocyte proliferation and hypertrophic differentiation. Dev Cell 2002;3:439–49.

92. Grimsrud CD, Romano PR, D'Souza M, et al. BMP signaling stimulates chondrocyte maturation and the expression of Indian hedgehog. J Orthop Res 2001;19:18–25.

93. Yoon BS, Pogue R, Ovchinnikov DA, et al. BMPs regulate multiple aspects of growth-plate chondrogenesis through opposing actions on FGF pathways. Development 2006;133:4667–78.

94. Rountree RB, Schoor M, Chen H, et al. BMP receptor signaling is required for postnatal maintenance of articular cartilage. PLoS Biol 2004;2: e355.

95. Klaus A, Birchmeier W. Wnt signalling and its impact on development and cancer. Nat Rev Cancer 2008;8:387–98.

96. Chen Y, Alman BA. Wnt pathway, an essential role in bone regeneration. J Cell Biochem 2009;106: 353–62.

97. Hartmann C, Tabin CJ. Dual roles of Wnt signaling during chondrogenesis in the chicken limb. Development 2000;127:3141–59.

98. Hartmann C, Tabin CJ. Wnt-14 plays a pivotal role in inducing synovial joint formation in the developing appendicular skeleton. Cell 2001;104: 341–51.

99. Spater D, Hill TP, Gruber M, et al. Role of canonical Wnt-signalling in joint formation. Eur Cell Mater 2006;12:71–80.

100. Dao DY, Yang X, Chen D, et al. Axin1 and Axin2 are regulated by TGF- and mediate cross-talk between TGF- and Wnt signaling pathways. Ann N Y Acad Sci 2007;1116:82–99.

101. Hill TP, Spater D, Taketo MM, et al. Canonical Wnt/beta-catenin signaling prevents osteoblasts from differentiating into chondrocytes. Dev Cell 2005;8: 727–38.

102. Church V, Nohno T, Linker C, et al. Wnt regulation of chondrocyte differentiation. J Cell Sci 2002;115: 4809–18.

103. Dong YF, Soung do Y, Schwarz EM, et al. Wnt induction of chondrocyte hypertrophy through the Runx2 transcription factor. J Cell Physiol 2006; 208:77–86.

104. Chun JS, Oh H, Yang S, et al. Wnt signaling in cartilage development and degeneration. BMB Rep 2008;41:485–94.

105. Ryu JH, Chun JS. Opposing roles of WNT-5A and WNT-11 in interleukin-1beta regulation of type II collagen expression in articular chondrocytes. J Biol Chem 2006;281:22039–47.

106. Kawakami Y, Tsuda M, Takahashi S, et al. Transcriptional coactivator PGC-1alpha regulates chondrogenesis via association with Sox9. Proc Natl Acad Sci U S A 2005;102:2414–9.

107. Chung UI. Essential role of hypertrophic chondrocytes in endochondral bone development. Endocr J 2004;51:19–24.

108. Zelzer E, Glotzer DJ, Hartmann C, et al. Tissue specific regulation of VEGF expression during bone development requires Cbfa1/Runx2. Mech Dev 2001;106:97–106.

109. de Crombrugghe B, Lefebvre V, Nakashima K. Regulatory mechanisms in the pathways of cartilage and bone formation. Curr Opin Cell Biol 2001;13:721–7.

110. Zelzer E, Olsen BR. The genetic basis for skeletal diseases. Nature 2003;423:343–8.

111. Poole AR. An introduction to the pathophysiology of osteoarthritis. Front Biosci 1999;4:D662–70.

112. Millan FA, Denhez F, Kondaiah P, et al. Embryonic gene expression patterns of TGF beta 1, beta 2 and beta 3 suggest different developmental functions in vivo. Development 1991;111:131–43.

113. Massague J, Seoane J, Wotton D. Smad transcription factors. Genes Dev 2005;19:2783–810.

114. Ballock RT, Heydemann A, Wakefield LM, et al. TGF-beta 1 prevents hypertrophy of epiphyseal chondrocytes: regulation of gene expression for cartilage matrix proteins and metalloproteases. Dev Biol 1993;158:414–29.

115. Bohme K, Winterhalter KH, Bruckner P. Terminal differentiation of chondrocytes in culture is a spontaneous process and is arrested by transforming growth factor-beta 2 and basic fibroblast growth factor in synergy. Exp Cell Res 1995;216:191–8.

116. Dieudonne SC, Semeins CM, Goei SW, et al. Opposite effects of osteogenic protein and transforming growth factor beta on chondrogenesis in cultured long bone rudiments. J Bone Miner Res 1994;9:771–80.

117. Iwai T, Murai J, Yoshikawa H, et al. Smad7 Inhibits chondrocyte differentiation at multiple steps during endochondral bone formation and down-regulates p38 MAPK pathways. J Biol Chem 2008;283:27154–64.

118. Day TF, Guo X, Garrett-Beal L, et al. Wnt/beta-catenin signaling in mesenchymal progenitors controls osteoblast and chondrocyte differentiation during vertebrate skeletogenesis. Dev Cell 2005;8:739–50.

119. Tamamura Y, Otani T, Kanatani N, et al. Developmental regulation of Wnt/beta-catenin signals is required for growth plate assembly, cartilage integrity, and endochondral ossification. J Biol Chem 2005;280:19185–95.

120. Gaur T, Rich L, Lengner CJ, et al. Secreted frizzled related protein 1 regulates Wnt signaling for BMP2 induced chondrocyte differentiation. J Cell Physiol 2006;208:87–96.

121. Bodine PV, Zhao W, Kharode YP, et al. The Wnt antagonist secreted frizzled-related protein-1 is a negative regulator of trabecular bone formation in adult mice. Mol Endocrinol 2004;18:1222–37.

122. Lane NE, Nevitt MC, Lui LY, et al. Wnt signaling antagonists are potential prognostic biomarkers for the progression of radiographic hip osteoarthritis in elderly Caucasian women. Arthritis Rheum 2007;56:3319–25.

123. Min JL, Meulenbelt I, Riyazi N, et al. Association of the Frizzled-related protein gene with symptomatic osteoarthritis at multiple sites. Arthritis Rheum 2005;52:1077–80.

124. Lamb R, Thomson W, Ogilvie E, et al. Wnt-1-inducible signaling pathway protein 3 and susceptibility to juvenile idiopathic arthritis. Arthritis Rheum 2005;52:3548–53.

125. Schett G, Zwerina J, David JP. The role of Wnt proteins in arthritis. Nat Clin Pract Rheumatol 2008;4:473–80.

126. Corr M. Wnt-beta-catenin signaling in the pathogenesis of osteoarthritis. Nat Clin Pract Rheumatol 2008;4:550–6.

127. Chen M, Zhu M, Awad H, et al. Inhibition of beta-catenin signaling causes defects in postnatal cartilage development. J Cell Sci 2008;121:1455–65.

128. Zhu M, Chen M, Zuscik M, et al. Inhibition of beta-catenin signaling in articular chondrocytes results in articular cartilage destruction. Arthritis Rheum 2008;58:2053–64.

129. Diarra D, Stolina M, Polzer K, et al. Dickkopf-1 is a master regulator of joint remodeling. Nat Med 2007;13:156–63.

130. Johnson ML, Kamel MA. The Wnt signaling pathway and bone metabolism. Curr Opin Rheumatol 2007;19:376–82.

131. Kubota T, Michigami T, Ozono K. Wnt signaling in bone metabolism. J Bone Miner Metab 2009;27:265–71.

132. Cawston TE, Wilson AJ. Understanding the role of tissue degrading enzymes and their inhibitors in development and disease. Best Pract Res Clin Rheumatol 2006;20:983–1002.

133. Inada M, Wang Y, Byrne MH, et al. Critical roles for collagenase-3 (Mmp13) in development of growth plate cartilage and in endochondral ossification. Proc Natl Acad Sci U S A 2004;101:17192–7.

Structural and Functional Maturation of Distal Femoral Cartilage and Bone During Postnatal Development and Growth in Humans and Mice

Elaine F. Chan, MS[a], Ricky Harjanto, BS[a],
Hiroshi Asahara, MD, PhD[d], Nozomu Inoue, MD, PhD[e,f],
Koichi Masuda, MD[c], William D. Bugbee, MD[g],
Gary S. Firestein, MD[b], Harish S. Hosalkar, MD[h],
Martin K. Lotz, MD[d], Robert L. Sah, MD, ScD[a,i],*

KEYWORDS

- Distal femur • Postnatal development • Growth strain
- Joint shape • Statistical shape modeling

The load-bearing and compositional properties of articular cartilage vary with both the size and shape of the diarthrodial joint. In skeletally mature animals and humans, the biomechanical and biochemical characteristics of articular cartilage vary by site (eg, patellofemoral groove vs femoral condyles) and joint (eg, knee vs ankle),[1–7] complementing the local geometry to respond to various

This work was supported by grants from the National Institutes of Health, the National Science Foundation, and the Howard Hughes Medical Institute through the HHMI Professors Program (to UCSD for R.L.S.). Additional individual support was received through NSF Graduate Fellowships (to E.F.C.) and UCSD Chancellor's Research scholarship (to R.H.). This project acknowledges the use of the Cornell Center for Advanced Computing's "MATLAB on the TeraGrid" experimental computing resource funded by NSF grant 0844032 in partnership with Purdue University, Dell, The MathWorks, and Microsoft.

[a] Department of Bioengineering, University of California—San Diego, 9500 Gilman Drive, La Jolla, CA 92093-0412, USA

[b] Department of Medicine, University of California—San Diego, 9500 Gilman Drive, La Jolla, CA 92093-0656, USA

[c] Department of Orthopedic Surgery, University of California—San Diego, 9500 Gilman Drive, La Jolla, CA 92093-0863, USA

[d] Department of Molecular and Experimental Medicine, Scripps Research Institute, 10550 North Torrey Pines Road, La Jolla, CA 92037-1000, USA

[e] Department of Biomedical Engineering, Doshisha University, 1-3 Tatara Miyakodani, Kyotanabe City, Kyoto 610-0394, Japan

[f] Department of Orthopedic Surgery, Rush University Medical Center, 1611 West Harrison Street, Chicago, IL 60612-3833, USA

[g] Division of Orthopedic Surgery, Scripps Clinic, 10666 North Torrey Pines Road, La Jolla, CA 92037, USA

[h] Department of Orthopedic Surgery, Rady Children's Hospital, 3030 Children's way, San Diego, CA 92123, USA

[i] Institute of Engineering in Medicine, University of California—San Diego, 9500 Gilman Drive, La Jolla, CA 92093, USA

* Corresponding author. Department of Bioengineering, University of California—San Diego, Mail Code 0412, 9500 Gilman Drive, La Jolla, CA 92093.
E-mail address: rsah@ucsd.edu

loading demands of the body. During postnatal development (the processes of differentiation and growth), joint size increases, and cartilage thickness and chondrocyte density decrease.[8–10] Concomitantly, articular cartilage load-bearing material properties improve. In animal knees, increases during development in the tensile and compressive moduli of articular cartilage have been associated with increases in collagen content and cross-linking.[6,7,11,12]

The macroscopic mechanisms that dictate cartilage material maturation and joint shaping remain to be determined. At the articular surface, appositional growth[13,14] occurs with chondrocyte proliferation in the superficial zone[15,16] and deposition of collagen fibers.[17] Articular cartilage maturation is also affected by changes at the bone-cartilage interface, with chondrocyte proliferation occurring in neonatal rabbit knee joints above the subchondral plate.[15,18] These macroscopic tissue changes during growth may be described biomechanically by growth deformations and strains.[19] Thinning of cartilage during postnatal development is due to mineralization in the deep zone and advancement of the tidemark, separating the deep and calcified cartilages. In conjunction with these axial growth processes, articular cartilage expands tangentially along with the underlying subchondral bone. Both axial and tangential growth processes may generate internal stresses[20] and affect the material quality of adult articular cartilage. Thus, a detailed understanding of the shape of the bone-cartilage interface during development would provide insight into the biomechanics of cartilage maturation and macroscopic joint size and shape.

The length and shape of long bones during in vivo development is in part contributed through the differential growth and remodeling of articular and growth plate cartilages. Both begin as a homogeneous condensation of chondrocytes that undergo proliferation, hypertrophy, and mineralization in distinct zones to form a highly organized structure at maturity.[10,21–26] In the growth plate, rates of chondrocyte proliferation, hypertrophy, and matrix production in different zones have been related to longitudinal bone growth.[26–29] Differences in these rates at specific locations give rise to differential elongation rates, such as those observed at opposite ends of long bones and between different joints. Additional variations in cartilage growth rates and directions with age and species produce the wide range of joint shapes and relative proportions of anatomic features (eg, lateral and medial condyle proportions in the knee).

Current knowledge of the macroscopic joint shape is based on measurements of cartilage and bone geometries from gross specimens, plain radiographs, magnetic resonance imaging (MRI), and computed tomography (CT). However, the complexities of joint shape are challenging to represent by 2-dimensional (2-D) or best-fit 3-dimensional (3-D) measurements.[30,31] While the distal femur is characterized by measurements such as anterior-posterior length, medial-lateral width, and intercondylar height,[32,33] these parameters are confounded by the size of the knee, especially in growing knees, making it difficult to distinguish shape changes during joint maturation. Statistical shape modeling (SSM)[34,35] is one technique that can concisely quantify complex shapes in a limited number of independent parameters based on a sample population. This method can automatically identify corresponding anatomic regions between samples with high reproducibility,[36] making it ideal for studying shape changes during growth and development. Both 2-D and 3-D SSMs have been used to analyze joint shape and bone density as risk factors for the development of osteoarthritis[36–42] and osteoporotic fractures,[43–45] but have yet to be applied to the growth of healthy joints.

The hypothesis of this study was that shape changes of the distal femur at the bone-cartilage interface vary differentially with age and anatomic region during postnatal growth and development. The aims were to (1) illustrate and qualitatively compare the shape changes of the bone-cartilage interface during normal development in humans and C57BL/6 wild-type mice, (2) establish a statistical shape model and determine shape parameters for the growth of the mouse distal femur from postnatal days 12 to 120, and (3) determine growth deformation and strain rates of the bone-cartilage interface. Quantification of the shape plasticity throughout growth and development provides the foundation for investigating in vivo developmental biomechanics of the knee. In addition, quantitative models of the developing knee are useful as design targets for tissue engineering that extends to the joint scale, as well as for the development of new technologies for the clinical diagnosis and treatment of skeletal disorders.

MATERIALS AND METHODS
Sample Preparation and Imaging

With Institutional Review Board approval, clinical CT scans were obtained from 6 patients (range: 3.9–11.9 years; mean: 8.2 years) with tibial torsion abnormalities but morphologically normal distal femora at 0.4 to 0.6 mm in-plane resolution and 0.63 mm slice thickness (GE Lightspeed VCT; GE Healthcare, Piscataway, NJ, USA).

The structure of mouse knee joints was assessed by micro–computed tomography (µCT) and histology. With Institutional Animal Care and Use Committee approval, both hindlimbs of 21 C57BL/6 male mice, n = 3 pairs each at 12, 16, 20, 24, 30, 60, and 120 days postnatal, were harvested, fixed in 10% neutral buffered formalin, and scanned intact by μCT at $(9 \ \mu m)^3$ isotropic voxel resolution (SkyScan 1076; SkyScan, Kontich, Belgium; 70 kVp, 140 μA, 1750 ms exposure). Following μCT, 1 femur at each age point was randomly selected for histologic processing. Proximal and distal femora were decalcified in 10% formic acid and paraffin-embedded. Sagittal sections (5 μm thick) were obtained approximately through the center of the medial femoral condyle of the distal femur. Sections were stained with Safranin-O and digitized at 20× magnification (0.5 μm resolution) with an Aperio ScanScope (Aperio Technologies, Vista, CA, USA).

Gross Morphology

Human and mouse CT images were qualitatively analyzed for morphologic changes at the bone-cartilage interface during developmental growth in 2-D coronal and sagittal planes through the center of the load-bearing region of the condyle and in 3-D reconstructions. Distal femora were assessed for contour of the condyles, posterior condyle prominence, medial femoral condyle (MFC) versus lateral femoral condyle (LFC) size, and trochlear ridge development, as well as location and morphology of the growth plate. Contour of the opposing tibial plateau, as well as joint space width between the distal femoral and proximal tibial secondary ossification centers (SOCs), were also noted.

Histology

Safranin-O sections were compared with matching μCT sections of mouse femora to interpret the bone-cartilage interface of the SOC relative to the overlying articular-epiphyseal cartilage. In addition, histology sections were assessed for chondrocyte hypertrophy and organization.

Image Processing

All CT and μCT scans were imported into Mimics (Materialise, Leuven, Belgium) for surface segmentation and 3-D reconstruction. Left femora were flipped in orientation to match right femora. Bone-cartilage interfaces were identified by thresholding for bone, segmented, and exported as point clouds.

Width and Thickness Measurements

Transepicondylar widths were determined in human and mouse distal femora as a measure of growth. In 3-D reconstructed models, transep-icondylar width was measured as the nearest distance from the edge of the lateral epicondyle to the edge of the medial epicondyle. In the mouse, the overall length of the femur was also determined from the most proximal point on the femoral head to the most distal point on the femoral condyles.

Thicknesses of the articular-epiphyseal and growth plate cartilage were calculated from 2-D histology images. Articular-epiphyseal cartilage was defined from the articular surface to the calcified cartilage tidemark, or to the distal edge of large hypertrophic cells for young joints with no tidemark. Growth plate cartilage was defined from the epiphyseal side of reserve zone chondrocytes to the metaphyseal side of terminal hypertrophic zone chondrocytes. Because articular-epiphyseal and growth plate cartilage contours were highly curved in the mouse distal femur, making it difficult to estimate thickness directly, cartilage thickness was calculated as the area of the cartilage divided by the average width of the cartilage.

Statistical Shape Modeling

Both femora of 15 mice, n = 3 pairs each at days 12, 24, 30, 60, and 120, were used as the initial training samples for SSM. Training samples were rigidly registered and isotropically scaled[46] to the largest femur (day 120 sample). Point-to-point correspondences between coordinates of each femur were defined automatically, following previously established methods[47] by first constructing a normalized average atlas shape and then extrapolating points (landmark coordinates), in corresponding locations to each femur. Each distal femur was described by 412 landmarks, located from the femoral condyles to the proximal edge of the trochlea.

The statistical shape model was built from the landmarks of the training samples using principal component analysis.[34,47] A mean shape was calculated from training sample landmarks, and deviations of each shape from the mean were determined. Singular value decomposition of the covariance matrix was performed to obtain the eigenvectors and corresponding eigenvalues (in descending order). The eigenvectors represent the modes of variation within the training set, analogous to the principal axes of an ellipse. The eigenvalues represent the variance explained by each mode, or the amount of contribution of each mode to overall joint shape variation. Using the modes of variation from the model, the shape parameters, b, of each sample was calculated by $X = \bar{X} + Pb$, where $\bar{X}$ is the mean shape, $P = (p_1 \ | \ p_2 \ | \ ... \ | \ p_t)$ are the first t modes of variation that explain greater than 90% of the total shape variance, and X is the sample shape. Shape parameters are analogous to principal radii of an ellipse. Parameters were normalized to 1 standard deviation of the mode, calculated as the square root of the corresponding eigenvalue.

Additional samples at days 16 and 20 were analyzed by applying the SSM. Samples were segmented in Mimics, rigidly aligned to the same reference femur from the training set, and non-rigidly aligned to the model atlas shape to extrapolate landmarks. Shape parameters were then determined as described above.

Growth Maps: Deformation Rates, Strain Rates, and Strain Directions

Deformation and principal surface strain rates between ages were calculated from corresponding landmark coordinates of the average shape at each age. Here, landmark coordinates represented non-scaled shapes. Samples were aligned at the centroid of the growth plate to determine deformations during growth. Magnitudes of deformation were calculated as the distance between corresponding landmarks, and deformations in the same direction as the outward surface normal vector were defined as positive. The 2-D components of Green's strain[48] E_{ij} were calculated from $ds^2 - ds_0^2 = 2E_{ij}dX_idX_j$ for i,j = 1:2, where $ds_0^2 = dX_idX_j$ is the squared segment length of a pair of landmarks at the first age point, and ds^2 is the squared length at the second age point. Maximum principal strain rates and directions were calculated from the Green strain components.[48]

Deformation and strain rates were mapped in 3-D onto the triangulated surfaces of the average shape at each age point. Surface patches intersecting the transverse plane and sagittal plane through the medial condyle were determined, and the 3-D principal strain directions of those patches were projected onto each plane to illustrate strain directions along the 2-D surface contour.

Statistics

Differences in mode parameters between age points were assessed by a one-way analysis of variance with post hoc Tukey test. All data are expressed as mean ± SD.

RESULTS
Gross Morphology of the Developing Distal Femur: Human and Mouse

The overall size and shape of both human (**Figs. 1**A and **2**A) and mouse (**Figs. 1**B and **2**B) distal femoral bone-cartilage interface changed markedly over the evaluated growth period, as visualized by μCT in coronal (**Fig. 1**a) and sagittal (**Fig. 1**b) planes, and in 3-D reconstructions (see **Fig. 2**).

In the human, the femoral growth plate was situated just proximal to the posterior edge of the condyles and was relatively flat in the transverse plane (**Figs. 1**A-b and **2**A-b, c). At age 4 years, femoral condyle contours were round in both coronal and sagittal planes (**Fig. 1**A-i). At age 7 years, the posterior condyle was prominent, and the sagittal contour became elliptical. The MFC appeared slightly larger than the LFC. By age 12 years, the load-bearing region of the femoral condyles flattened in the coronal plane, whereas the sagittal profile remained elliptical (**Fig. 1**A-iii). A prominent intercondylar notch was observed in the coronal view. Extension of the lateral trochlear ridge was evident at 7 years and was prominent by 12 years (**Fig. 2**A-a). As the lateral trochlea developed, the lateral side of the growth plate became larger than the medial side (**Fig. 2**A-b). Joint space width between femoral and tibial epiphyseal bone decreased noticeably with age (**Fig. 1**A-a). At the opposing joint surface, proximal tibia SOC was round at age 4 years, developed flat plateaus by age 7 years, and had concave plateaus by age 12 years (see **Fig. 1**A-a).

In the mouse, growth plates were also situated proximal to the posterior edge of the condyle but had an undulating shape in the transverse plane, with 4 regions that extended convex toward the articular surface (**Fig. 2**B-b, c). At postnatal day 12 (**Fig. 1**B-ib), the femoral SOC had a rounded distal contour and an undulating proximal contour matching the growth plate geometry. Between days 16 and 24, SOCs expanded radially as femoral condyles extended outward, and the geometry of the epiphysis interlocked with the metaphysis (**Fig. 1**B-ii). At day 30, the posterior condyle became prominent, and the load-bearing regions of the condyles were flattened in the coronal plane (**Fig. 1**B-iii). The MFC also extended more medially compared with the LFC. By day 60, the shape of the knee had stabilized. Prominence of the lateral trochlear ridge, an evolutionary feature of bipedalism,[49] was not observed in mice. Similar to humans, joint space width between femoral and tibial epiphyseal bone decreased with age (**Fig. 1**B-a). In contrast to humans, mouse growth plates remained approximately symmetric in the medial-lateral direction throughout development (see **Fig. 2**B-b). Proximal tibial SOCs were rounded at day 12, flattened with 2 plateaus at day 20, concave toward the distal femur at day 30, and fully developed by day 60 (see **Fig. 1**B-a).

Rapid joint-scale growth occurred from age 4 to 12 years in the human and during the first 30 days in mice. Transepicondylar width in the

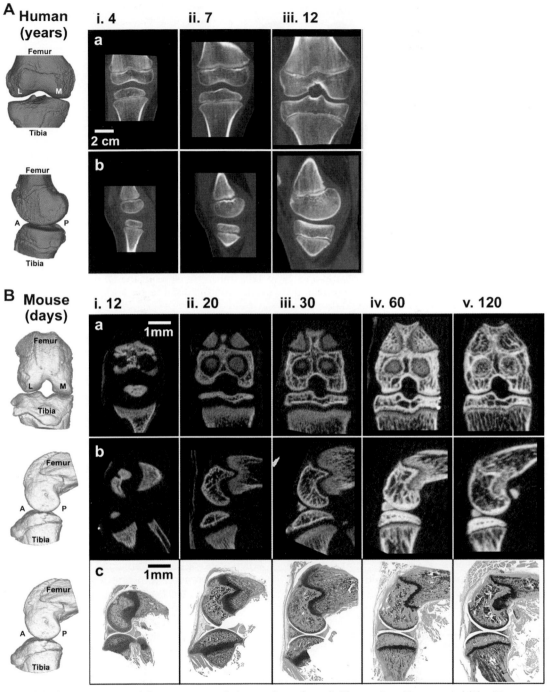

Fig. 1. (*A*) Clinical CT scans of the asymptomatic human knee from (*i–iii*) ages 4 to 12 years, and (*B*) μCT scans and Safranin-O sections of C57BL/6 wild-type mouse knees from (*i–v*) postnatal days 12 to 120, in (*a*) coronal and (*b, c*) sagittal views. A, anterior; L, lateral; M, medial; P, posterior.

human distal femur (**Fig. 3**A) increased linearly from age 4 to 12 (R^2 = 0.95; 4 years, 45.3 mm; 12 years, 78.9 mm), whereas transepicondylar width in the mouse femur (**Fig. 3**B) increased up to day 30, after which it plateaued (12 days, 1.9 mm; 30 days, 2.7 mm; 120 days, 2.8 mm). Overall femur length in the mouse increased at a slower pace and did not plateau until day 60 (**Fig. 3**C). Femur length at day 12 was approximately 50% that of day 120. The final length and volume of the mouse femur at day 120 were 15.2 ± 0.2 mm and 47.0 ± 4.3 mm^3, respectively.

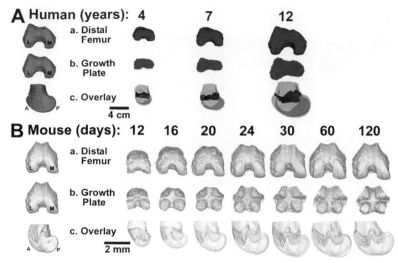

Fig. 2. 3-D reconstructions of the developing right distal femur and growth plate (*A*) in the human from ages 4 to 12 years, and (*B*) in the mouse from postnatal days 12 to 120. Transverse views of the (*a*) distal femur and (*b*) growth plate, and (*c*) sagittal views of the growth plate overlaid on the distal femur are shown. A, anterior; L, lateral; M, medial; P, posterior.

Histology

In C57BL/6 mice, both articular-epiphyseal and growth plate cartilage stained intensely with Safranin-O at all ages, with zonal and age-associated variations in cellular organization (see **Fig. 1**B-c; **Fig. 4**).

At day 12, articular-epiphyseal cartilage regions contained randomly distributed chondrocytes, with large hypertrophic chondrocytes at the SOC (see **Fig. 4**A-i). By day 30, the zonal architecture of articular cartilage was apparent with underlying bone formation, and by day 60 the articular cartilage was fully formed with a continuous subchondral bone plate.

Growth plate cartilage exhibited a distinct architecture with reserve, proliferative, and hypertrophic zones that decreased in height with age (see **Fig. 4**-ii). At day 12, hypertrophic chondrocytes in the articular-epiphyseal complex that stained with Safranin-O were not visible on μCT (see **Figs. 1**B-b, c, and **4**A). At day 20, bony regions in histology sections corresponded well with mineralized regions observed on μCT, and proliferative zone chondrocyte nuclei stained prominently (see **Fig. 4**B). By day 60, hypertrophic chondrocytes were essentially absent from the growth plate (see **Fig. 4**D).

Articular-epiphyseal and growth plate cartilage of the opposing proximal tibia showed similar age-dependent patterns of cellular organization and matrix staining (see **Fig. 4**-iii).

Cartilage Thickness

Articular-epiphyseal cartilage thickness in the mouse decreased with age and plateaued after day 60 (**Fig. 5**). Thickness measurements from

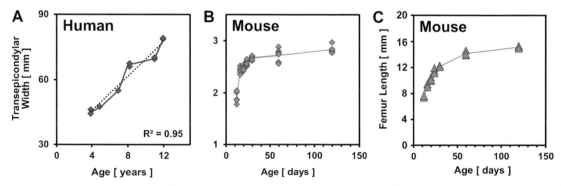

Fig. 3. Transepicondylar width of (*A*) human and (*B*) mouse distal femur, and (*C*) mouse femur length, measured in 3-D reconstructions of individual samples.

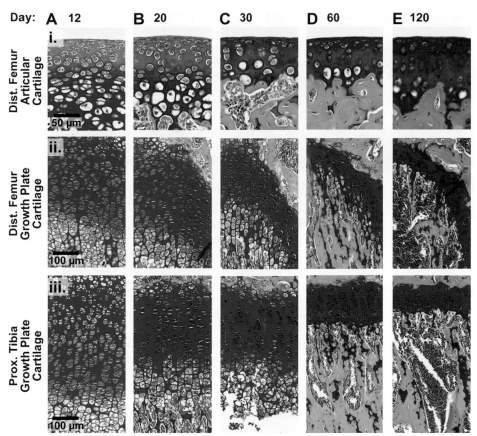

Fig. 4. Safranin-O sections of mouse distal femoral (*i*) articular-epiphyseal cartilage, (*ii*) growth plate cartilage, and proximal tibial (*iii*) growth plate cartilage showing distinct patterns of cellular organization at postnatal days (*A*) 12, (*B*) 20, (*C*) 30, (*D*) 60, and (*E*) 120. Images are oriented such that the articular surface is at the top.

histology at days 12 and 120 were 0.17 mm and 0.03 mm, respectively. Growth plate cartilage thickness also decreased with age and did not plateau by day 120. Growth plate cartilage thickness at days 12 and 120 was 0.56 mm and 0.10 mm, respectively. Both articular-epiphyseal and growth plate cartilage thickness were inversely correlated with overall femur length (articular-epiphyseal cartilage, $R^2 = 0.93$; growth plate cartilage, $R^2 = 0.94$).

Statistical Shape Model: Mouse Distal Femoral Bone-Cartilage Interface

In size-normalized data, 11 modes of variation accounted for greater than 90% of the total shape variation during developmental growth of the distal femur. The first 5 modes of variation accounted for 83% of total shape variation and described mid-condyle outward extension, posterior condyle upward extension, the relative size and medial extension of the MFC, varus/valgus rotation, and trochlea protrusion and intercondylar notch width, respectively (**Fig. 6**). Modes 6 to 11 accounted for 7% of the total shape variation, and described minor shape changes of the condyles and trochlear groove.

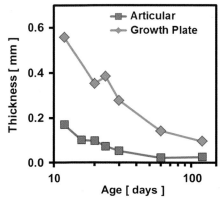

Fig. 5. Articular-epiphyseal and growth plate cartilage thickness in C57BL/6 wild-type mice with age, determined in 2-D histology sections.

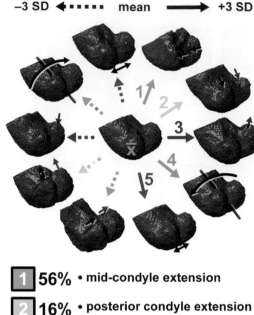

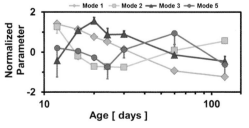

1 **56%** • mid-condyle extension

2 **16%** • posterior condyle extension

3 **6%** • relative size of MFC

4 **2%** • varus/valgus rotation

5 **2%** • intercondylar notch width

Fig. 6. First 5 modes of variation of the distal femur of CB57BL/6 mice. Colored solid/dashed lines indicate ±3 standard deviations from the mean. Black lines depict major changes in shape.

Shape parameters for Modes 1, 2, 3, and 5 were significantly different between age points in the distal femur (**Fig. 7**, **Table 1**; $P<.01$). From days 12 to 60, the femoral condyles underwent mid-condyle extension (decrease in Mode 1 parameter from 1.42 to −0.93), after which Mode 1 parameters plateaued. The posterior condyle region extended outward from day 12 to day 30 (decrease in Mode 2 parameter from 1.25 to −0.76), then retracted relative to the rest of the

Fig. 7. Normalized parameters for Modes of Variation 1, 2, 3, and 5 as a function of age. Data are shown as mean ± SD.

distal femur up to day 120. The relative size of the MFC (Mode 3 parameter) peaked at day 20, and slowly decreased up to day 120. Intercondylar notch width (Mode 5 parameter) widened from days 12 to 24, then became narrow up until day 60, and widened again at day 120.

Mode 1 parameters, describing mid-condyle extension, were linearly correlated with femur length, articular-epiphyseal cartilage thickness, and growth-plate cartilage thickness ($R^2 = 0.96$, 0.83, and 0.94, respectively).

Growth Maps: Deformation Rates, Strain Rates, and Strain Directions

Deformation and surface growth strains per day in the distal femur were highest at the condyles at day 12 and decreased with time (**Figs. 8** and **9**). Deformation rates were 0.14 mm per day between days 12 and 16, and decreased to <0.01 mm per day between days 60 and 120. Between days 16 and 20, strain rates were higher in the MFC than in the LFC, with maximum strains of 0.12 per day. Between days 20 and 24, strain rates were highest on the medial side of the LFC and the intercondylar notch, and between days 24 and 30 on the lateral side of the MFC. After day 30, strain rates were small (<0.03 per day). Regions of maximum strain corresponded well with regions of high deformation.

In general, directions of maximum strain were similar between all ages in the transverse and sagittal planes (**Fig. 10**). Strain directions in the transverse plane between days 12 and 16 were most variable, with strains in both directions along the surface contour. Along both sides of the epicondyles, directions of maximum strain primarily pointed up toward the trochlea (see **Fig. 10**A). At the load-bearing surface of the medial condyle, principal strains were directed medially. Strain directions in the lateral condyle were more variable, with direction vectors pointing medial and lateral between days 12 and 30, and lateral after day 30. In the sagittal plane (see **Fig. 10**B), a distinct transition point was visible near the center of the load-bearing surface of the MFC (and LFC, not shown) at all ages, where strains posterior to this location pointed toward the posterior condyle, and strains anterior to the location pointed anteriorly toward the trochlea. Surface strains of the trochlea pointed proximally, away from the condyles.

DISCUSSION

Development of the distal femoral bone-cartilage interface was generally similar between humans and mice, with subtle differences in condyle and trochlea morphology between the 2 species (see

Table 1
Distal femur mode parameters at different age points (mean ± SD)

Age (days)	Mode of Variation				
	1	2	3	4	5
12	1.42 ± 0.13	1.25 ± 0.31	−0.42 ± 0.59	−0.02 ± 0.70	0.21 ± 1.45
16	1.14 ± 0.07	−0.21 ± 0.17	1.08 ± 0.09	−0.27 ± 0.46	0.06 ± 0.13
20	0.77 ± 0.08	−0.71 ± 0.09	1.55 ± 0.18	0.74 ± 0.35	−0.26 ± 0.15
24	0.53 ± 0.05	−0.73 ± 0.14	0.88 ± 0.31	0.18 ± 0.52	−0.73 ± 0.60
30	0.15 ± 0.07	−0.76 ± 0.04	0.90 ± 0.17	−0.18 ± 0.78	0.13 ± 0.41
60	−0.93 ± 0.11	0.09 ± 0.26	−0.14 ± 0.53	−0.65 ± 1.42	0.95 ± 0.86
120	−1.23 ± 0.10	0.56 ± 0.13	−0.45 ± 0.24	0.67 ± 1.16	−0.62 ± 0.56
% Variance explained	56.5	15.7	6.5	2.3	2.1

Figs. 1–3). Distal femur size increased linearly up to age 12 years in humans and day 30 in mice, with transepicondylar widths of 79 mm and 2.7 mm, respectively. In both species, the distal femoral SOC began with a rounded contour, followed by protrusion of the condyles and trochlear ridges and the appearance of the intercondylar notch. Using SSM, it was possible to represent these intricate and complex 3-D size and shape changes with 11 modes of variation and corresponding shape parameters (see **Figs. 6** and **7**). From day 12, mouse mid-condyles extended outward up to day 60, associated with a decrease in Mode 1 parameter from 1.42 to −0.93, as posterior condyle regions extended up to day 30 and then partially retracted (Mode 2, **Fig. 7**). Concomitantly, the relative size and medial extension of the MFC increased and peaked at day 24 (Mode 3), with related trends in intercondylar notch width (Mode 5). Mode 1 shape parameters (mid-condyle extension) were highly correlated with overall femur length and the thickness of articular-epiphyseal and growth plate cartilages (see **Fig. 5**). In addition, growth deformations and strains decreased with age and were consistent with shape parameters (see **Figs. 8–10**). Principal strain directions demonstrated that trochlear and shaft strains pointed proximally while a sharp transition point in strain directions existed at the center

of the MFC load-bearing region. Together, these results quantitatively illustrate how the bone-cartilage interface takes form and expands during postnatal development and growth.

As with all animal and modeling studies, several limitations exist in the study design and interpretation of results. Quantitative assessment of shape changes during development was performed with wild-type C57BL/6 mice, a commonly used laboratory strain. The ages chosen for this study cover the range of mouse development starting from the appearance of the SOC as detectable by μCT, to puberty (~30 days), skeletal maturity (~60 days), and up to early adulthood.[50–52] Human development was observed up to puberty (age 12 years) for comparison. Although inherent differences in anatomy exist between humans and mice, trends in the model are applicable to human development since both species undergo the same general sequence of development that leads to functional adaptation and skeletal maturity. In the growth model, statistical shape analysis was used to describe shape-related variations of the mouse distal femur, normalized for joint size. As such, shape parameters from the model quantified relative, and not absolute, changes in proportions of anatomical features. In addition, surface strain rates between ages were calculated by assuming an exact anatomical correspondence

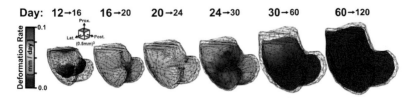

Fig. 8. Distal femoral shape at days 12, 16, 20, 24, 30, 60, and 120. Color maps on the younger shape indicate deformation rates (mm per day), calculated between the age intervals indicated at the top. Distal femoral shape at the older age point is overlaid (outline) for comparison.

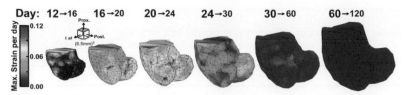

Fig. 9. Distal femoral shape at days 12, 16, 20, 24, 30, and 60. Color maps indicate maximum principal strain rates (per day), calculated between the age intervals indicated at the top and mapped onto the shape of the younger age point.

between landmark coordinates of samples extrapolated during SSM (extrapolation precision was within 0.03 mm).

The growth and attainment of shape in the distal femur was similar in humans and mice, even with substantial differences in growth plate morphology. Transepicondylar width increased in humans from age 4 years up to puberty, comparable with that of mice between days 12 and 30 (see **Fig. 3**), and was observed to plateau similarly after puberty.[53] In both species, femoral condyles developed from a rounded contour in sagittal and coronal planes to elliptical and flattened contours (see **Figs. 1** and **2**). As condyle shape and relative proportions of the MFC to LFC changed, growth plate morphology did not vary noticeably, supporting the theory that growth plates primarily contribute to longitudinal bone growth while radial expansion of the SOC affects joint shape, with final shape modulated by biomechanical loading.[17,26,54,55] However, lateral extension of the human growth plate occurred in conjunction with prominence of the lateral trochlear ridge, suggesting that the distal femoral growth plate may have a role in dictating trochlear morphology. The observed similarities and differences between human and mouse bone-cartilage interfaces serve as a basis for the interpretation and generalization of the results of SSM.

This study is the first to quantitatively describe shape variations, normalized for size, throughout postnatal development in MFC/LFC proportion, extension of the condyles, and intercondylar notch width. The plateau of shape parameters at ~60 days in mice corresponded well with the cessation of femur growth, finalization of zonal organization in articular-epiphyseal and growth plate cartilage, and stabilization of distal femur geometry (see **Figs. 1–4** and **7**). However, during the rapid lengthening phase, the distal femur underwent variations in shape that were not directly related to femur length and chondrocyte organization. Extension of the posterior condyle peaked around day 20 and decreased afterward, similar to the relative size of the MFC. By contrast, intercondylar notch width widened from days 12 to 20, narrowed up to day 60, and became wider again at day 120. It is unclear how functional adaptation or preprogrammed differential growth played a role in defining these transient shapes. One of the most striking changes during pediatric skeletal development in humans is the reorientation of the tibiofemoral angle from greater than 15° varus at birth to 10° valgus around 3 years of age, and finally decreasing to approximately 6° valgus by 6 to 7 years of age, with associated growth of the MFC.[56,57] Similar angular remodeling changes in the mouse may be related to the observed variations in MFC size and shape described here. Analysis of these transient developmental shapes may also provide insight into questions such as why certain intercondylar

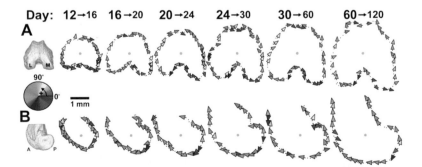

Fig. 10. Directions of maximum strain (corresponding to strain rates shown in **Fig. 9**) across the right distal femur (*A*) transverse plane and (*B*) sagittal plane through the medial condyle. Direction vectors were calculated between age intervals indicated at the top and mapped onto the shape of the younger age point. Orientation and color of arrowhead indicate direction of the vector with respect to the horizontal axis. Gray dots are points of reference at corresponding locations. A, anterior; L, lateral; M, medial; P, posterior.

notch shapes predispose the joint to osteoarthritis in adults,[58] but not in adolescents.

This study also is the first to provide a direct estimate of growth deformation and strain vectors. Growth maps highlighted the spatially distinct shape changes throughout development and corresponded well with shape parameters. As deformation and strain rates were higher in the MFC than in the LFC between days 16 and 20, Mode 3 parameters for relative MFC size peaked (large MFC/LFC size), and as rates were high on the medial side of the LFC between days 20 and 24, Mode 5 parameters for notch width decreased (narrow width). The alternating patterns of higher growth rates on the MFC and LFC surfaces are reminiscent of adaptive shaping of the femoral condyles as the body responds to internal and external factors. Temporal and joint-specific variations during growth and development have previously been observed in the dynamics of collagen remodeling[59–61] and biomechanics of articular cartilage.[6,7,11,62] However, little is known about the spatial distribution of matrix components during growth in the knee, especially between the MFC and LFC. It would be interesting in future studies to investigate the relationship between developmental shape changes within the MFC and LFC, and the properties of articular cartilage in those regions of highest change.

Principal strain directions in the transverse and sagittal planes illustrated directional patterns of growth that have previously only been assumed or qualitatively described.[63] The general pattern of principal directions remained fairly consistent between ages, even as strain rates decreased with age. One interesting finding from this study was the distinct transition point in principal directions located within the load-bearing region of the condyle in the sagittal view (see **Fig. 10**B). This location may be the central point of mid-condyle growth and extension, as surface strains around it were directed in opposite directions. Strains on the sides of the epicondyles in the transverse view were directed up toward the trochlea (see **Fig. 10**A), which may be related to the emergence of trochlear ridges. Along the load-bearing regions of the MFC in the transverse view, strains were directed medially, matching the medial extension and growth of the MFC as described by the shape parameters (see **Figs. 7** and **10**A). These unique strain-direction patterns of the developing distal femur serve as snapshots in time through which in vivo joint development and the mechanisms behind cartilage structural maturation can be better understood.

In conclusion, this study characterized the macroscopic shape and in vivo growth strains of the distal femur at the bone-cartilage interface throughout postnatal growth. Comparisons between human and mouse provided a qualitative assessment of the morphologic differences between species and insight into the evolutionary mechanisms of joint development. SSM and resultant parameters quantitatively defined initial, final, and transient geometries of the mouse distal femur during growth. The first 5 modes of variation accounted for the shapes of major anatomic features such as the condyles and intercondylar notch, whereas latter modes were associated with fine-tuning of positions and curvatures within the joint. Growth deformation and strain maps showed highest rates in the femoral condyles and strain direction vectors that corresponded with the emergence of anatomic features. Accurate quantification of the bone-cartilage interface geometry is imperative for furthering the understanding of macroscopic mechanisms of cartilage maturation and overall joint development, as well as for developing new technologies for the diagnosis and treatment of joint disorders.

REFERENCES

1. Maroudas A, Evans H, Almeida L. Cartilage of the hip joint: topographical variation of glycosaminoglycan content in normal and fibrillated tissue. Ann Rheum Dis 1973;32:1–9.
2. Kiviranta I, Tammi M, Jurvelin J, et al. Topographical variation of glycosaminoglycan content and cartilage thickness in canine knee (stifle) joint cartilage: application of the microspectrophotometric method. J Anat 1987;150:265–76.
3. Armstrong SJ, Read RA, Price R. Topographical variation within the articular cartilage and subchondral bone of the normal ovine knee joint: a histological approach. Osteoarthritis Cartilage 1995;5:25–33.
4. Jurvelin JS, Arokoski JP, Hunziker EB, et al. Topographical variation of the elastic properties of articular cartilage in the canine knee. J Biomech 2000; 33:669–75.
5. Treppo S, Koepp H, Quan EC, et al. Comparison of biomechanical and biochemical properties of cartilage from human knee and ankle pairs. J Orthop Res 2000;18:739–48.
6. Williamson AK, Chen AC, Sah RL. Compressive properties and function-composition relationships of developing bovine articular cartilage. J Orthop Res 2001;19:1113–21.
7. Williamson AK, Chen AC, Masuda K, et al. Tensile mechanical properties of bovine articular cartilage: variations with growth and relationships to collagen network components. J Orthop Res 2003;21:872–80.

8. Schenk RK, Eggli PS, Hunziker EB. Articular cartilage morphology. In: Kuettner K, Schleyerbach R, Hascall VC, editors. Articular cartilage biochemistry. New York: Raven Press; 1986. p. 3–22.

9. Eggli PS, Hunziker EB, Schenk RK. Quantitation of structural features characterizing weight- and less-weight-bearing regions in articular cartilage: a stereological analysis of medial femoral condyles in young adult rabbits. Anat Rec 1988;222:217–27.

10. Jadin KD, Bae WC, Schumacher BL, et al. Three-dimensional (3-D) imaging of chondrocytes in articular cartilage: growth-associated changes in cell organization. Biomaterials 2007;28:230–9.

11. Julkunen P, Harjula T, Iivarinen J, et al. Biomechanical, biochemical and structural correlations in immature and mature rabbit articular cartilage. Osteoarthritis Cartilage 2009;17:1628–38.

12. Wong M, Ponticiello M, Kovanen V, et al. Volumetric changes of articular cartilage during stress relaxation in unconfined compression. J Biomech 2000; 33:1049–54.

13. Archer CW, Morrison H, Pitsillides AA. Cellular aspects of the development of diarthrodial joints and articular cartilage. J Anat 1994;184:447–56.

14. Hayes AJ, MacPherson S, Morrison H, et al. The development of articular cartilage: evidence for an appositional growth mechanism. Anat Embryol (Berl) 2001;203:469–79.

15. Mankin HJ. Localization of tritiated thymidine in articular cartilage of rabbits. I. growth in immature cartilage. J Bone Joint Surg Am 1962;44:682–98.

16. Oreja MR, Quintáns Rodriguez M, Abelleira AC, et al. Variation in articular cartilage in rabbits between weeks six and eight. Anat Rec 1995;241:34–8.

17. Hunziker EB, Kapfinger E, Geiss J. The structural architecture of adult mammalian articular cartilage evolves by a synchronized process of tissue resorption and neoformation during postnatal development. Osteoarthritis Cartilage 2007;15:403–13.

18. Mankin HJ. Localization of tritiated thymidine in articular cartilage of rabbits. III. mature articular cartilage. J Bone Joint Surg Am 1963;45:529–40.

19. Cowin SC. Tissue growth and remodeling. Annu Rev Biomed Eng 2004;6:77–107.

20. Klisch SM, Chen SS, Sah RL, et al. A growth mixture theory for cartilage with applications to growth-related experiments on cartilage explants. J Biomech Eng 2003;125:169–79.

21. Stockwell RA, Meachim G. The chondrocytes. In: Freeman MA, editor. Adult articular cartilage. 2nd edition. Tunbridge Wells (England): Pitman Medical; 1979. p. 69–144.

22. Hunziker EB, Quinn TM, Hauselmann HJ. Quantitative structural organization of normal adult human articular cartilage. Osteoarthritis Cartilage 2002;10:564–72.

23. Schumacher BL, Su JL, Lindley KM, et al. Horizontally oriented clusters of multiple chondrons in the superficial zone of ankle, but not knee articular cartilage. Anat Rec 2002;266:241–8.

24. Jadin KD, Wong BL, Bae WC, et al. Depth-varying density and organization of chondrocyte in immature and mature bovine articular cartilage assessed by 3-D imaging and analysis. J Histochem Cytochem 2005;53:1109–19.

25. Hunziker EB. Growth plate structure and function. Pathol Immunopathol Res 1988;7:9–13.

26. Wilsman NJ, Farnum CE, Leiferman EM, et al. Differential growth by growth plates as a function of multiple parameters of chondrocytic kinetics. J Orthop Res 1996;14:927–36.

27. Farnum CE, Wilsman NJ. Determination of proliferative characteristics of growth plate chondrocytes by labeling with bromodeoxyuridine. Calcif Tissue Int 1993;52:110–9.

28. Wilsman NJ, Farnum CE, Green EM, et al. Cell cycle analysis of proliferative zone chondrocytes in growth plates elongating at different rates. J Orthop Res 1996;14:562–72.

29. Hunziker EB. Mechanism of longitudinal bone growth and its regulation by growth plate chondrocytes. Microsc Res Tech 1994;28:505–19.

30. Than P, Sillinger T, Kranicz J, et al. Radiographic parameters of the hip joint from birth to adolescence. Pediatr Radiol 2004;34:237–44.

31. Hitt K, Shurman JR 2nd, Greene K, et al. Anthropometric measurements of the human knee: correlation to the sizing of current knee arthroplasty systems. J Bone Joint Surg Am 2003;85(Suppl 4):115–22.

32. Lonner JH, Jasko JG, Thomas BS. Anthropomorphic differences between the distal femora of men and women. Clin Orthop Relat Res 2008;466:2724–9.

33. Mahfouz M, Abdel Fatah EE, Bowers LS, et al. Three-dimensional morphology of the knee reveals ethnic differences. Clin Orthop Relat Res 2012;470:172–85.

34. Cootes TF, Taylor CJ, Cooper DH, et al. Active shape models—their training and application. Comput Vis Image Understand 1995;61:38–59.

35. Hamarneh G, Abu-Gharbieh R, Gustavsson T. Review. Active shape models—part I: modeling shape and gray level variation. Uppsala (Sweden): Swedish Symposium on Image Analysis;1998.

36. Williams TG, Holmes AP, Waterton JC, et al. Anatomically corresponded regional analysis of cartilage in asymptomatic and osteoarthritic knees by statistical shape modelling of the bone. IEEE Trans Med Imaging 2010;29:1541–59.

37. Gregory JS, Waarsing JH, Day J, et al. Early identification of radiographic osteoarthritis of the hip using an active shape model to quantify changes in bone morphometric features: can hip shape tell us anything about the progression of osteoarthritis? Arthritis Rheum 2007;56:3634–43.

38. Lynch JA, Parimi N, Chaganti RK, et al. The association of proximal femoral shape and incident

radiographic hip OA in elderly women. Osteoarthritis Cartilage 2009;17:1313–8.

39. Waarsing JH, Rozendaal RM, Verhaar JA, et al. A statistical model of shape and density of the proximal femur in relation to radiological and clinical OA of the hip. Osteoarthritis Cartilage 2010;18:787–94.

40. Waarsing J, Kloppenburg M, Slagboom P, et al. Osteoarthritis susceptibility genes influence the association between hip morphology and osteoarthritis. Arthritis Rheum 2011;63(5):1349–54.

41. Bredbenner TL, Eliason TD, Potter RS, et al. Statistical shape modeling describes variation in tibia and femur surface geometry between Control and Incidence groups from the osteoarthritis initiative database. J Biomech 2010;43:1780–6.

42. Shepstone L, Rogers J, Kirwan J, et al. The shape of the distal femur: a palaeopathological comparison of eburnated and non-eburnated femora. Ann Rheum Dis 1999;58:72–8.

43. Baker-Lepain JC, Luker KR, Lynch JA, et al. Active shape modeling of the hip in prediction of incident hip fracture. J Bone Miner Res 2011;26(3):468–74.

44. Nicolella DP, Bredbenner TL. Development of a parametric finite element model of the proximal femur using statistical shape and density modelling. Comput Methods Biomech Biomed Engin 2012;15(2):101–10.

45. Gregory JS, Testi D, Stewart A, et al. A method for assessment of the shape of the proximal femur and its relationship to osteoporotic hip fracture. Osteoporos Int 2004;15:5–11.

46. Myronenko A, Song X. Point-set registration: Coherent Point Drift. IEEE Trans Pattern Anal Mach Intell 2010;32:2262–75.

47. Frangi A, Niessen W, Rueckert D, et al. Automatic 3D ASM construction via atlas-based landmarking and volumetric elastic registration. Information processing in medical imaging lecture notes in computer science, 2001, vol 2082/2001. p. 78–91.

48. Fung YC. A first course in continuum mechanics. 2nd edition. Englewood Cliffs (NJ): Prentice-Hall; 1977.

49. Tardieu C, Glard Y, Garron E, et al. Relationship between formation of the femoral bicondylar angle and trochlear shape: independence of diaphyseal and epiphyseal growth. Am J Phys Anthropol 2006;130:491–500.

50. Serrat MA, Lovejoy CO, King D. Age- and site-specific decline in insulin-like growth factor-I receptor expression is correlated with differential growth plate activity in the mouse hindlimb. Anat Rec (Hoboken) 2007;290:375–81.

51. Kilborn SH, Trudel G, Uhthoff H. Review of growth plate closure compared with age at sexual maturity and lifespan in laboratory animals. Contemp Top Lab Anim Sci 2002;41:21–6.

52. Zoetis T, Tassinari MS, Bagi C, et al. Species comparison of postnatal bone growth and development. Birth Defects Res B Dev Reprod Toxicol 2003;68:86–110.

53. Griffin FM, Math K, Scuderi GR, et al. Anatomy of the epicondyles of the distal femur: MRI analysis of normal knees. J Arthroplasty 2000;15:354–9.

54. Sissons HA, Kember NF. Longitudinal bone growth of the human femur. Postgrad Med J 1977;53:433–7.

55. Hall BK. Fins into limbs: evolution, development, and transformation. Chicago: University of Chicago Press; 2007.

56. Shapiro F. Pediatric orthopedic deformities. San Diego (CA): Academic Press; 2001.

57. Salenius P, Vankka E. The development of the tibio-femoral angle in children. J Bone Joint Surg Am 1975;57:259–61.

58. Shepstone L, Rogers J, Kirwan JR, et al. Shape of the intercondylar notch of the human femur: a comparison of osteoarthritic and non-osteoarthritic bones from a skeletal sample. Ann Rheum Dis 2001;60:968–73.

59. Bank RA, Bayliss MT, Lafeber FP, et al. Ageing and zonal variation in post-translational modification of collagen in normal human articular cartilage. The age-related increase in non-enzymatic glycation affects biomechanical properties of cartilage. Biochem J 1998;330:345–51.

60. Keene DR, Oxford JT, Morris NP. Ultrastructural localization of collagen types II, IX, and XI in the growth plate of human rib and fetal bovine epiphyseal cartilage: type XI collagen is restricted to thin fibrils. J Histochem Cytochem 1995;43:967–79.

61. van Turnhout MC, Schipper H, Engel B, et al. Postnatal development of collagen structure in ovine articular cartilage. BMC Dev Biol 2010;10:62.

62. Brommer H, Brama PA, Laasanen MS, et al. Functional adaptation of articular cartilage from birth to maturity under the influence of loading: a biomechanical analysis. Equine Vet J 2005;37:148–54.

63. Tardieu C. Short adolescence in early hominids: infantile and adolescent growth of the human femur. Am J Phys Anthropol 1998;107:163–78.

Effect of Exercise on Articular Cartilage

Harpal K. Gahunia, MSc, PhD[a],*,
Kenneth P.H. Pritzker, MD, FRCPC[b,c,d]

KEYWORDS

- Articular cartilage • Exercise • Biomechanics • Aging

Joints are composed of specialized connective tissues which, from a functional point of view, act synergistically to effectively and efficiently deal with the mechanical loads encountered over a lifetime.[1,2] When performing various tasks such as standing, walking or running, the knee frequently encounters forces up to several magnitudes higher than body weight.[3–5]

Articular cartilage plays a crucial role in maintaining mechanical competence by providing an almost frictionless gliding surface of synovial joints. Under physiologic conditions, knee cartilage has the unique capability to withstand hydrostatic pressure and the ability to uniformly transmit and dissipate enormous forces across the joint from one subchondral bone to the other during motion. These cartilage features are due to its molecular composition and 3-dimensional architecture, coupled with its highly hydrated state and biomechanical properties.[1,2,6–11] As such, articular cartilage has the ability to withstand high compressive forces associated with not only activities of daily living but also activities with markedly increased locomotive stresses such as sports. However, the ability of the cartilage to perform its biomechanical functions can be compromised by changes in tissue properties that occur with normal aging, injury, or diseases such as chondromalacia patella, osteochondritis dissecans, osteoarthritis (OA), and rheumatoid arthritis.

Traditionally, the effects of exercise on articular cartilage have been examined in animal models, and little information was available on human cartilage. Recent improvements in magnetic resonance imaging (MRI) technology has allowed visualization of human articular cartilage *in vivo* enabling researchers to investigate the variations in the morphologic and biochemical components of human knee articular cartilage during loading and compressive forces while exercising as well as in diseased states.[12–14]

Physical exercise, performed frequently over time, has been shown to increase bone and muscle mass (eg, body building), whereas states of inactivity or microgravity have been associated with tissue atrophy.[15,16] The biosynthetic activity of chondrocytes has also been experimentally shown to be regulated by mechanical stimuli.[17,18] Based on these *in vitro* findings, mathematical models have been developed that explain the variable thickness of cartilage between joints based on differences in mechanical loading magnitude.[19–22] Current findings suggest that the human cartilage deforms very little *in vivo* during physiologic activities and recovers from deformation within 90 minutes after loading.[12,13]

Several studies have shown that with immobilization cartilage undergoes atrophy when subjected to reduced loading conditions and that cartilage thickness is only partially restored with exercise.[23–29] Both clinical and animal research have shown that continuous passive motion of the joint, after joint procedures, is an important stimulus for articular cartilage regeneration.[30–32]

The authors have no conflicts of interest to disclose.

[a] Orthopedic Science Consulting Services, Oakville, Ontario, Canada
[b] Department of Laboratory Medicine and Pathobiology, University of Toronto, Toronto, Ontario, Canada
[c] Department of Surgery, University of Toronto, Toronto, Ontario, Canada
[d] Pathology and Laboratory Medicine, Mount Sinai Hospital, 600 University Avenue, Toronto, Ontario, Canada, M5G 1X5
* Corresponding author.
E-mail address: harpal.gahunia@utoronto.ca

Orthop Clin N Am 43 (2012) 187–199
doi:10.1016/j.ocl.2012.03.001

Cartilage adapts to mechanical stimuli by altering its morphology, 3-D architecture, and composition (proteoglycan, collagen, and interstitial water content). This article reviews the structural and biochemical composition of articular cartilage and the macroenvironment and microenvironment of chondrocytes. Also summarized are the effects of exercise on articular cartilage macromolecular synthesis and degradation as well as the extent to which the level of exercise would result in beneficial effects on normal and injured knee cartilage.

ARTICULAR CARTILAGE

Articular cartilage is a highly specialized connective tissue with biophysical properties consistent with its ability to withstand high compressive forces. The biochemical properties and organization of the macromolecular constituents of the cartilage matrix and their interaction with water molecules is the key to the shock-absorbing property of the tissue.

During growth and development of long bones (a period from fetal development to cessation of bone growth), articular cartilage goes through a series of structural, morphologic, and biochemical changes. Adult cartilage is typically avascular, alymphatic, and aneural.[33] As such, nourishment is provided through long-range diffusion of the joint fluid. Until the epiphyseal plate is fully ossified in childhood, the articular cartilage is capable of receiving some nutrition through diffusion of substances from blood vessels in the subchondral bone.[34] The unique biological and mechanical properties of articular cartilage depend on the cartilage architecture and the interactions between the extracellular matrix (ECM) and the chondrocytes that maintain the cartilage function.[9]

CHONDRONS

Chondrons are the microanatomical, micromechanical, and metabolically active functional units of articular cartilage. Anatomically, a chondron comprises the chondrocyte and its pericellular microenvironment.[35–37] Morphologically, a transparent pericellular glycocalyx is present on the chondrocyte surface and is enclosed by a fibrillar pericellular capsule containing type VI collagen.[38,39] The composition and structural integrity of the chondron pericellular microenvironment have been shown to influence the chondrocytic response to experimental osmotic challenge.[38] The chondron plays an important role *in vivo* to maintain the homeostasis of the articular cartilage and to mediate the chondrocytic response to physicochemical changes of the cartilage macromolecules and the movement of water and ions within the matrix.[36,38] Thus, chondron acts hydrodynamically to protect the integrity of the chondrocyte and its pericellular microenvironment during compressive loading.

Throughout life, the articular cartilage undergoes continual internal remodeling. Chondrocytes can synthesize and secrete the cartilage macromolecular components and can also degrade the matrix by releasing degradative enzymes, such as collagenase, and other metalloproteinases, including stromelysin. During growth and development, synthesis outweighs the degradation. In adults, matrix synthesis is finely balanced by controlled matrix degradation.[40,41] Hence, chondrocytes continually replace the matrix macromolecules lost during normal degradation. However, disruption to the normal balance of synthesis and degradation can lead to variation in the intrinsic characteristics of the cartilage zones, resulting in a gradual degeneration of the ECM that is responsible for the development of clinically recognizable diseases.[42,43]

CARTILAGE EXTRACELLULAR MATRIX

The ECM of cartilage (95% cartilage volume) is a resilient gel comprising 60% to 80% (cartilage wet weight) tissue fluid with a complex macromolecular organization consisting mainly of type II collagen and proteoglycans, which in humans represent 55% and 35% of cartilage dry weight, respectively.[44] Evidence exists that there are interactions between proteoglycan aggregates and collagen fibers and that collagen-proteoglycan binding increases with age.[45–48] The intrinsic physical properties of collagen fibers (relatively insoluble with high tensile strength) and proteoglycan (soluble with high fixed charge density and compressive rigidity) primarily determine the biomechanical properties of cartilage. The compressive properties of articular cartilage are a function of the balance between the osmotic swelling generated by water bound to the sulfate and carboxylate groups of the proteoglycan and the tension developed in the collagen network surrounding the proteoglycan. The noncollagenous proteins in cartilage ECM include fibronectin, anchorin, tenascin, cartilage oligomeric matrix protein, and cartilage matrix glycoprotein.[49–52]

ARTICULAR CARTILAGE COLLAGENS

Five genetically distinct collagen types are known to exist in adult articular cartilage. Type II collagen (90%–95% of the total cartilage collagen types) is the major structural protein in cartilage and is also essentially unique to cartilaginous tissues.[53-55] Through its high tensile strength, type II collagen provides the structural integrity and resiliency to articular cartilage.[53,54,56-58] Type XI collagen, a fibril-forming collagen, contributes to about 2% to 3% of the total collagen and is incorporated in the type II collagen fiber in a ratio of about 1:30 in mature tissues.[55] Type XI collagen is thought to mediate physical interactions between collagen fibrils and proteoglycans in cartilage and to regulate the size of the type II collagen fibers.[59,60] Type IX collagen represents 1% to 2% of collagen in adult cartilage and at least 10% in fetal cartilage. Majority of type IX collagen is covalently cross-linked to the surface of type II collagen fibril. Type IX collagen is also distributed in the ECM without association with type II collagen.[61-63] Type IX collagen contains chondroitin sulfate or dermatan sulfate glycosaminoglycan side chains, which are thought to stabilize type II collagen fibril structure.[61,64] Type VI collagen, a short-helix molecule concentrated pericellularly that represents 1% to 2% of the total collagen, helps mediate the attachment of chondrocytes to the macromolecular framework of the matrix.[65,66] Type X collagen (1%), a short nonfibrillar collagen present adjacent to hypertrophied chondrocytes and in the calcified zone, is thought to play an important role in the development of the growth plate and cartilage calcification.[67-70]

Collagen fibrils are stabilized by covalent cross-links formed between adjacent collagen chains (intramolecular cross-link) and adjacent collagen molecules (intermolecular cross-link). The tensile strength of the collagen fibers is dependent on the formation of intramolecular cross-links. Pyridinoline cross-links are abundant in cartilage collagen, and their concentration remains relatively constant with age.[71-74]

PROTEOGLYCANS

Proteoglycans are strongly hydrophilic, thus providing the lubrication and shock-absorbing property (resistance to compression) of articular cartilage. Proteoglycans are composed of a protein core onto which 1 or more glycosaminoglycan chains are covalently bonded. The glycosaminoglycan molecules are unbranched chains of repeating disaccharides. Hyaluronic acid is the only glycosaminoglycan that is not bound to a core protein and is nonsulfated. The heterogeneity of proteoglycan structure is a reflection of variation not only in the protein core but also in the type and size of the glycosaminoglycan chains. Variation in the position of sulfation can also increase diversity in the chemical and physical properties of the glycosaminoglycan chains. The glycosaminoglycan groups present in cartilage proteoglycan are primarily chondroitin sulfate (87%), which exists both as chondroitin-4-sulfate and chondroitin-6-sulfate, as well as keratan sulfate (6%) and hyaluronic acid. In articular cartilage, large aggregating proteoglycans (aggrecan and versican) form 50% to 58% of total proteoglycans, whereas large nonaggregating proteoglycans form 40% of total proteoglycans.[75] The relative concentration of glycosaminoglycan varies markedly with age. In immature cartilage, there is a preponderance of chondroitin-4-sulfate and little keratan sulfate. With advancing age, there is an appreciable increase in keratan sulfate content and a corresponding decrease in chondroitin-4-sulfate.[76]

NONCOLLAGENOUS PROTEINS

Small noncollagenous proteins and glycoproteins present in the cartilage ECM are thought to modulate several fibril properties.[77] Although glycoproteins form a small fraction (2%–5%) of the cartilage ECM, they play an important role in matrix assembly and/or regulation of matrix metabolism. Cartilage oligomeric matrix protein, a 524-kDa glycoprotein, is found in cartilage during chondrogenesis. It is preferentially localized in the territorial matrix surrounding the chondrocytes.[50,78] Biglycan, decorin, and fibromodulin are members of a family of structurally related proteoglycan. They bind to the ECM macromolecules and help to stabilize the matrix. Biglycan, a 100-kDa molecule with a core protein of 38 kDa, is localized in the pericellular matrix.[79] Decorin, a 74-kDa proteoglycan with a core protein of 36 kDa, is present throughout the interterritorial ECM with increased amounts in the superficial zone of articular cartilage, is thought to mediate interactions between aggrecans and collagens.[80-82] Fibromodulin (59 kDa), a small collagen-binding proteoglycan, is abundant on cartilage surface adjacent to the bursae. Fibronectin is a glycoprotein of the ECM that participates in matrix assembly and affects cell adhesion, morphology, migration, and differentiation.[83,84] Fibronectin plays an important role in the adhesion of chondrocytes to ECM and is implicated in tissue repair.[85] Tenascin, an oligomeric glycoprotein, functions in processes such as wound repair and cartilage formation and is thought to influence interactions between the chondrocytes and the cartilage matrix.

Cartilage matrix glycoprotein (molecular weight = 54 kDa) is a major component of the cartilage ECM, which is thought to bind and bridge type II collagen fibrils.[86,87] Matrix Gla protein is a vitamin

K–dependent 10-kDa protein that is known to inhibit cartilage calcification. Anchorin CII (31-kDa noncollagenous protein) mediates in anchoring chondrocytes with type II collagen,[88,89] whereas chondronectin specifically mediates the attachment of chondrocytes to type II collagen.[90] Link protein (molecular weight = 45 kDa) binds to both cartilage aggrecan and hyaluronic acid in ECM, thereby stabilizing their aggregation.[91]

CARTILAGE MATRIX COMPARTMENTALIZATION

Articular cartilage consists of morphologically distinct zones that serve varied functions, including the formation of an articulating surface and a compression-resistant core as well as its attachment to the bone. The uncalcified cartilage can be distinguished microscopically into 3 zones, which are parallel to and extend from the articular surface to the tidemark. The differences between the zones are based on chondrocyte morphology and distribution, collagen and proteoglycan composition/concentration, collagen architecture, and water content. The uncalcified articular cartilage is attached to the subchondral bone via a narrow layer of calcified cartilage. In adults, a densely basophilic calcified line called the tidemark demarcates the interface between uncalcified and calcified cartilage.[92,93]

The superficial zone forming the cartilage surface adjacent to the synovial space is characterized by small ellipsoid chondrocytes with their long axis parallel to the articular surface. The collagen fibers are densely packed and orientated parallel to the articular surface. The middle zone consists of large, round, and randomly distributed chondrocytes with gothic arch-like architecture of collagen fibers.[94] The deep zone consists of large chondrocytes arranged in longitudinal columns that are oriented perpendicular to the articular surface and with radially oriented collagen fibers. The calcified zone is characterized by small chondrocytes embedded in a heavily calcified matrix.[95,96]

In immature cartilage, the distinction between the middle zone and deep zone is less apparent. The cells just beneath the superficial zone have proliferative activity.[97] This activity ceases with maturity, but all chondrocytes continue to have latent capacity to proliferate and regenerate matrix. Cellularity is considerably reduced during development, especially in the deep zone.[98] In immature cartilage, proteoglycan content is least in the middle zone compared with the articular and deep (epiphyseal) zones. Whereas the superficial zone of the mature cartilage has the highest collagen content and lowest proteoglycan content, the middle zone has the lowest collagen content.[99–101]

Matrix compartmentalization studies have revealed a clear subdivision of the middle and deep zones into pericellular, territorial, and interterritorial matrices.[37,102] Each chondrocyte cell membrane is immediately surrounded by pericellular (or lacunar) matrix, which is characterized by the absence of fibrillar collagen and abundance of proteoglycan. The pericellular matrix is composed of a mixture of hyaluronan, sulfated proteoglycans, biglycan, glycoproteins, fibronectin, laminin, and collagen type VI and IX.[49,103–106] Encapsulating the pericellular matrix is the territorial (or capsular) matrix, characterized by a fine network of fibrillar collagen.[107,108] The chondrocytes establish contact with these collagen fibrils by extending fine cytoplasmic processes. Adjacent to this is the outermost matrix compartment, the interterritorial region, which constitutes the largest domain of the matrix and lies in the space between various territorial matrices. The interterritorial matrix is characterized by collagen fibers interspersed with varying concentrations of proteoglycans, depending on the zone in which the chondrocytes lie.

AGING OF ARTICULAR CARTILAGE

Aging is associated with changes in the biochemical activity of the chondrocytes resulting in alterations in the ECM composition and decreased ability of articular cartilage to withstand compressive forces. This in turn could accelerate the cartilage degradation. Mitrovic and colleagues[96] documented age-related decrease in cell density in all zones of the human femoral condyle articular cartilage, although more markedly in the superficial zone.[96] Vascularity of the cartilage calcified zone (a sign of remodeling) is well developed after 55 to 65 years of age. Reduction in the cartilage fluid content from 70% to 80% (normal cartilage wet weight) to 50% to 65% accompanies the aging process, especially in the deeper zone.[109] Using bovine patella articular cartilage (with intact surfaces) from immature, mature, through to mildly degenerated tissue, Broom and colleagues showed a consistent pattern of increased free swelling of the isolated cartilage matrix with age and degeneration.[110] In humans, with aging, the knee cartilage is especially susceptible to becoming worn down and weakened, given the loads it is subjected over the years. Because of age-related changes in cartilage fluid and macromolecular content, structure, and architecture, the capability of articular cartilage to withstand compressive forces also decreases with aging.

EFFECT OF PHYSICAL ACTIVITY ON ARTICULAR CARTILAGE AND ADJACENT TISSUES

Joint exercise not only increases the blood flow to the various connective tissues of the joint but also keeps the joints lubricated. Consistent low to moderate daily activity facilitates cycles of catabolism and anabolism within these tissues. When breakdown and repair are well balanced, homeostasis of joint tissues is maintained. However, a drastic increase or decrease in the intensity of the physical activity results in homeostatic imbalance. Often, after long periods of immobility, the joints become stiff and lose some of their range of movement. As such, strengthening of the knee tissues through regular exercise is of paramount importance.

Articular cartilage resides within the joint interior, and its health is dependent to a large extent on the integrity of other components such as the synovium, muscle, ligaments, tendons, and bone. Exercise has a number of effects on the skeletal system, both in the short and the long term. However, injuries due to extreme or improper exercise can not only affect the bone, muscle, ligament, or tendon but also unfavorably affect the articular cartilage, causing joint swelling, pain, and stiffness. Frequent movement of the joints can relieve the symptoms of pain due to increased circulation of tissue fluid in the joints. Weight-bearing exercise such as walking, jogging or running has several benefits, including improved blood circulation and decreased tissue fluid stagnation in a given joint area. Synovial fluid produced by the synovial membrane within the joints has a short-term response to exercise, thus requiring regular exercise to stay lubricated, nourished, and healthy.[111]

Several studies have alluded to the significant effects of exercise on the bones, muscles, tendons, ligaments, and cartilage of the skeletal system. Weight-bearing exercises, such as strength training and running, can stress long bones. In response to this stress, the osteoblasts build new bone, specifically at the sites of stimulus, resulting in greater bone density that is more capable of withstanding the impact when consistently stimulated. The bone is continuously resorbed and remodeled in response to external mechanical loads. However, excessive weight-bearing exercise without sufficient recovery results in greater breakdown than rebuilding ratio and could eventually contribute to stress fractures or osteoporosis. As such, high-impact exercise may cause harm to bones and other joint tissues due to high level of mechanical stress.[112] Likewise, too little weight-bearing exercise will not provide a stimulus for bone building and lead to overall bone loss.

Increases in sports performance such as marathon running can be at least partly attributed to strengthening of connective tissue components of the joint as well as adaptations in muscle, although the cellular mechanisms underlying these adaptations remain unclear. Of the skeletal tissues, muscle responds most rapidly to exercise. The muscles used in the particular exercise rebuild themselves by synthesizing more muscle proteins and increasing in size. Consistent exercising of these muscles is necessary to maintain this size increase. Without adequate stimulation via exercise, the particular muscles will experience an accelerated catabolic activity resulting in muscle atrophy as observed during the extended period of immobilization or non–weight bearing after knee surgery.

The integrity of tendons and ligaments is critical for skeletal system function. Because tendons and ligaments connect bones to muscles and bones to bones, respectively, they facilitate coordinated movement by transmitting force across the joints. When exposed to regular exercise, ligaments become stronger and more resistant to injury. Because ligaments have limited blood supply, adaptations of any kind are slow to develop. A study on the effect of certain types of exercise on ligaments and tendons revealed that the cross-sectional area of both structures increases in response to running and other load-bearing activities and conversely decreases during periods of immobilization postsurgery.[113] Tendons and ligaments are bundles of collagen-containing fibers that transmit muscle force across the joint. Consistent stimulation through exercise increases the size, density, and number of collagen fibers making up tendons and ligaments. In addition, a stronger muscle transmits more force through the tendon, increasing its strength over time.

Articular cartilage is a highly hydrated specialized connective tissue with the capability to withstand impact forces. The therapeutic value of exercise to cartilage is now known. Regular exercise facilitates diffusion of nutrients through the cartilage, and moderate exercise likely improves the molecular composition of cartilage. Too little exercise or immobilization eventually compromises the lubricant properties of cartilage, although this can be reversed with more activity. However, too much loading on the cartilage at the joints can lead to OA, characterized by excessive cartilage breakdown and eventual cartilage loss.[114]

Research on the effects of exercise on cartilage has shown that similar to bone, cartilage tends to weaken without regular loading.[115,116] However, unlike bone, cartilage does not actually appear to thicken even in highly active people such as elite athletes, although studies contradicting this observation exist. Researchers agree that vast differences in cartilage thickness between individuals exist, but what remains unclear is whether exercise is a significant contributor to this finding. Using MRI to accurately measure cartilage thickness during loading, Gratzke and colleagues[117] showed that direct measurements of muscle forces do not predict cartilage thickness more accurately than muscle cross-sectional areas. Their findings suggested that relative to muscle thickness, cartilage thickness has much less ability to adapt to mechanical loading.

JOINT ARTHROPATHY AND EFFECT OF EXERCISE

Exercise is important for healthy individuals as well as for people with conditions such as chondromalacia patella and arthritis and in those who have had a surgical procedure involving the knee joint. Studies have shown that maintaining healthy weight and keeping joint tissues strong through regular exercise is beneficial for patients with the above-mentioned conditions.

Chondromalacia patella is a term used to describe softening of the articular cartilage on the underside of the patella. Chondromalacia can occur by simple wear and tear on the knee joint or arthritis as people age. In young individuals, especially those who are actively involved in sports, chondromalacia is most likely a consequence of an acute injury such as a traumatic fall, repetitive overuse, knee malalignment, or even muscle weakness. This injury is common in runners, skiers, cyclists, and soccer players. Frequently, chondromalacia is associated with a dull pain under or around the patella that increases while walking downstairs or climbing upstairs as well as sitting or getting out of a chair. Low-impact exercise for chondromalacia strengthens the muscles, particularly the inner part of the quadriceps. Swimming, stationary bicycle, and cross-country skiing are good ways to strengthen the joint with minimal impact.

OA is the leading cause of disability among adults, resulting in knee pain, swelling, and stiffness. With increasing age, the "sponginess and cushioning" ability of cartilage is subject to degeneration due to wear, a process that can be exacerbated by previous injury, resulting in OA. Exercise is one of the most effective ways to reduce pain and improve function in patients with knee OA. Strength training as well as low-impact exercises such as cycling, tai chi, and swimming can also reduce pain in the knee affected by OA.

Based on the erroneous wear-and-tear concept of OA, the commonly held myth is that exercise will aggravate cartilage loss. However, with the advancement of MRI technology, Roos and colleagues[114] were able to determine the impact of moderate exercise on the knee cartilage of subjects at high risk for developing OA. This 4-month, randomized controlled trial was aimed to investigate the effects of moderate exercise in 45 patients (29 men and 16 women; age 35–50 years) with partial medial meniscus resection 3 to 5 years before the study period.[114] Subjects were randomly assigned to either an exercise group or a control group. The exercise group was enrolled in a supervised program of aerobic and weight-bearing exercise, for 1 hour, 3 times weekly for 4 months. At the study's onset and follow-up, subjects from both groups underwent MRI scans to evaluate knee cartilage morphology and glycosaminoglycan content. Subjects also answered a series of questions regarding their knee pain and stiffness, as well as their general activity level. In the exercise group, many subjects reported improvements in physical activity and functional performance tests compared with subjects in the control group. Their study showed that moderate exercise in these patients not only improved the joint symptoms and function but also increased the cartilage glycosaminoglycan content.[114] The investigators corroborated previous findings that supported the therapeutic value of exercise for patients with OA, for improving not only joint symptoms and function but also the quality of knee cartilage as seen on MRI. This implies that human cartilage responds to physiologic loading in a way similar to that exhibited by muscle and bone and that previously established positive symptomatic effects of exercise in patients with OA may occur in parallel or may even be caused by improved cartilage properties.

Another study, by Racunica and colleagues,[118] investigated the effect of physical activity with varying degrees of intensity, frequency, and duration on the knee cartilage and bone. A total of 297 healthy adults (aged 50–79 years), with no history of knee injury or OA, were recruited for the study. All the individuals underwent MRI examinations of the tibiofemoral joints of their dominant knee. Dominant knee was defined as the knee pertaining to the leg they first step forward when walking. MRI was used to assess cartilage and bone marrow lesions and to measure cartilage volume. Subjects answered specific questions regarding their exercise and walking habits, as well as routine activity at home and at work, to determine their level of physical activity at 6 months and 7 days before the study. Baseline data on body weight, height, body mass index, and physical activity were obtained for each subject. The increase in tibial cartilage volume correlated positively with the frequency and duration of vigorous activity. Also, moderate physical activity, including regular walking, was associated with a lower incidence of bone marrow lesions, indicating more resistance to fracture in the subchondral bone. The study by Racunica and colleagues demonstrated a protective effect of vigorous physical activity on knee cartilage in healthy adults and strongly supports the benefits of exercise for individuals at risk for OA. However, this study contradicts previous reports suggesting that high-level exercise is damaging to cartilage.

CARTILAGE-STRENGTHENING PHYSICAL ACTIVITY

Walking, using a treadmill or static bicycle helps to build strength in all the knee tissues, including articular cartilage. Stretching and strengthening the knee is important for any workout routine, in particular exercises that enhance the range of motion. Running, jumping, and other weight-bearing activities put the bones under stress, which forces the bones to respond by becoming stronger, whereas low-impact exercise, such as biking or swimming, puts little strain on the bones. Running, jumping, and other high-impact activities during childhood benefit cartilage and bone homeostasis by increasing the size and strength of the growing skeleton. Although weight-bearing exercises, including weight lifting and high-impact activities such as jumping or tumbling of gymnastics, increase muscle mass and bone density in young children, these activities may pose a risk of cartilage injury in the long term.[119–122] The risk of focal cartilage lesions and development of premature OA with repetitive high impact activities have also been reported in animal studies.[123–125]

Regular physical activity by individuals may strengthen their knee cartilage. Although walking downhill is usually tolerated well by healthy people, overuse may cause damage to the cartilage under the patella. Water aerobics is a way to perform normal activities without experiencing the impact of working out on land. Water workouts can involve aerobics, walking, or jogging. Cycling is another low-impact exercise that can stimulate the cartilage within joints.

Fat mass, such as in obese individuals, affects bones differently than muscle mass. A study involving 768 men (aged 25–45 years) suggested that bone size is adapted to the dynamic load imposed by muscle force rather than passive loading by fat.[126] However, the same principle does not apply to articular cartilage because long-term, repetitive, intense loading on cartilage has proved harmful to the tissue.

Following an 18-month clinical trial of diet and exercise, data were obtained from 142 overweight and obese adults older than 60 years, all of whom were diagnosed with knee OA and placed on weight loss programs to investigate the relationship between change in body mass and knee forces during walking. The results indicated that for every pound of weight lost, there was a 4-pound reduction in the load on the knee per step during daily activities.[127] The findings suggest that for obese individuals a loss of 10 pounds could translate to a decrease of 48,000 pounds in compressive loads per mile of walking that each knee is subjected to, which is a clinically relevant decrease.

Due to aging, repetitive high-impact or excessive exercise among adults may place the joint at risk for arthritis. A recent study showed that middle-aged men and women who engage in high levels of physical activity could damage their knee cartilage and increase their risk for OA.[112] The study involved men and women of healthy weight, without pain or other symptoms. Knee injuries were more common and more severe among those who engaged in the highest levels of physical activity.[112,128] High-impact, weight-bearing activities such as running and jumping can carry a greater risk of cartilage injury over long term. On the other hand, low-impact activities, such as swimming and cycling, may protect diseased adult cartilage from progressive degeneration. A study by Stehling and colleagues[112] involved 136 women and 100 men, aged 45 to 55 years, within a healthy weight range. The participants were separated into low-, middle-, and high-activity groups based on their level of physical activities. A person whose activity level was classified as high typically engaged in several hours of walking, sports, or other types of exercise per week.[112] MRI scans of study participants' knees were obtained to assess the tissues of the knee joint. Results showed that people in the high-activity group had cartilage and ligament lesions as well as bone marrow edema compared with those in the low-activity group. Also, the cartilage damage was 3 times more severe in the high-activity group. The participants' age or sex did not affect their risk of knee injury.[112]

High-impact activity, such as running for longer than 1 hour per day at least 3 times a week could be associated with cartilage degeneration and a higher risk for developing OA.[129] On the other hand, engaging in light exercise and refraining from frequent knee-bending activities may protect against the onset of the disease. Hovis and colleagues[129] recruited 132 asymptomatic participants at risk for knee OA, as well as 33 age-matched and body mass index–matched controls. Study participants (99 women and 66 men; ages, 45–55 years) were separated into 3 exercise and strength-training levels, based on their responses to the Physical Activity Scale for the Elderly questionnaire. Exercise levels included sedentary, light exercisers, and moderate to strenuous exercisers; strength-training groups included none, minimal, and frequent. Knee-bending activities were also analyzed. MRI examinations revealed that light exercisers had the healthiest knee cartilage among all exercise levels, and patients with minimal strength training had healthier cartilage than patients with either no strength training or frequent strength training.[129] Moderate to strenuous exercise in women was associated with higher water content and more degenerated collagen architecture in the knee cartilage. The results of this study indicate that moderate to strenuous exercise may accelerate cartilage degeneration, putting these women at even greater risk of developing OA. In addition, the findings showed that frequent knee-bending activities, such as climbing up at least 10 flights of stairs a day, lifting objects weighing more than 25 pounds, or squatting, kneeling, or deep knee bending for at least 30 minutes per day, were associated with higher water content and cartilage abnormalities.

SUMMARY

Age-associated and degenerative loss of functional integrity in articular cartilage develops from effects of cumulative and subtle changes in its extracellular matrix. Although articular cartilage appears to display atrophic changes during unloading and may exhibit compositional changes (increase in GAG) after exercise, it seems to differ from other musculoskeletal tissues with load-bearing function.[130–132] Whereas 'more' muscle provides more tensile strength, and 'more' bone provides higher structural compressive and bending strength and hence better protection against fractures, 'more' cartilage is not known to be associated with improved mechanical competence of joints. Hydrostatic pressurization provides a mechanism by which cartilage is able to distribute joint forces evenly onto the subchondral bone to protect itself from mechanical damage.[133–135]

Physical activity among children has been shown to have beneficial effects on knee cartilage.[136,137] Studies involving randomly selected healthy children without knee pain or injury showed increased cartilage volume (by 22% to 25%) among those involved in vigorous activity compared to mildly active children. In general, immature cartilage has a greater tolerance for vigorous physical activity compared to the adult knee cartilage. Adult cartilage is more susceptible to cartilage lesions with high-impact exercise level. These findings suggest that with aging, the level of physical activity has variable effect on knee cartilage. Known risk factors for cartilage degeneration include excess body weight, knee injuries, frequent knee bending and long-term severe or strenuous physical activity. Individuals can reduce their risk for OA by maintaining a healthy body weight and avoiding strenuous exercise. Long-term, lower-impact activities such as walking, swimming or using an elliptical trainer are likely more beneficial in terms of cartilage health than higher impact activities such as running or tennis.

Both human and animal studies have shown beneficial effect of exercise on subchondral bone mineral density.[125,138–140] These studies have illustrated that habitual low-intensity loading elicits a greater response in the subchondral bone mineral density relative to occasional high-intensity loading. During skeletal growth, regular weight-bearing exercise has beneficial effects on bone mineral content and density. Further, moderate physical activity and high-impact sports participation among athletic children have shown beneficial effects on bone (enhanced bone formation at the load-bearing sites) and muscle mass. Recent studies have illustrated the beneficial effects of exercise (low to moderate impact) on articular cartilage and its correlation with the biochemical changes that occur during compressive forces associated with physical activity.[114,129,141,142] However, the morphological and biochemical response of cartilage to exercise during growth through various stages of cartilage maturity have not been investigated. Given the complexity of the articular cartilage macromolecular and micromolecular three-dimensional architecture, several questions pertaining to the exercise duration, intensity and frequency remain unresolved. Also, further research is required to identify the types of activity that will optimize cartilage structure and biomechanical function during growth and development. This research may also shed light on the nature of optimal postsurgical rehabilitation to enhance the outcome of cartilage repair strategies in both young and adult patients.

REFERENCES

1. Ateshian GA, Wang H. A theoretical solution for the frictionless rolling contact of cylindrical biphasic

articular cartilage layers. J Biomech 1995;28(11): 1341–55.

2. Cohen ZA, Mow VC, Henry JH, et al. Templates of the cartilage layers of the patellofemoral joint and their use in the assessment of osteoarthritic cartilage damage. Osteoarthr Cartil 2003;11(8):569–79.

3. Liemohn W. Exercise and arthritis. Exercise and the back. Rheum Dis Clin North Am 1990;16(4): 945–70.

4. Ounpuu S. The biomechanics of running: a kinematic and kinetic analysis. Instr Course Lect 1990;39:305–18.

5. Wu G, Ladin Z. Limitations of quasi-static estimation of human joint loading during locomotion. Med Biol Eng Comput 1996;34(6):472–6.

6. Huang CY, Soltz MA, Kopacz M, et al. Experimental verification of the roles of intrinsic matrix viscoelasticity and tension-compression nonlinearity in the biphasic response of cartilage. J Biomech Eng 2003;125(1):84–93.

7. Huang CY, Stankiewicz A, Ateshian GA, et al. Anisotropy, inhomogeneity, and tension-compression nonlinearity of human glenohumeral cartilage in finite deformation. J Biomech 2005;38(4): 799–809.

8. Mow VC, Ateshian GA, Spilker RL. Biomechanics of diarthrodial joints: a review of twenty years of progress. J Biomech Eng 1993;115(4B):460–7.

9. Buckwalter JA, Mankin HJ. Articular cartilage: tissue design and chondrocyte-matrix interactions. Instr Course Lect 1998;47:477–86.

10. Hunziker EB, Quinn TM, Hauselmann HJ. Quantitative structural organization of normal adult human articular cartilage. Osteoarthr Cartil 2002;10(7): 564–72.

11. Mankin HJ, Thrasher AZ. Water content and binding in normal and osteoarthritic human cartilage. J Bone Joint Surg Am 1975;57(1):76–80.

12. Eckstein F, Hudelmaier M, Putz R. The effects of exercise on human articular cartilage. J Anat 2006;208(4):491–512.

13. Eckstein F, Lemberger B, Gratzke C, et al. In vivo cartilage deformation after different types of activity and its dependence on physical training status. Ann Rheum Dis 2005;64(2):291–5.

14. Mosher TJ, Liu Y, Torok CM. Functional cartilage MRI T2 mapping: evaluating the effect of age and training on knee cartilage response to running. Osteoarthr Cartil 2010;18(3):358–64.

15. Keller TS, Strauss AM, Szpalski M. Prevention of bone loss and muscle atrophy during manned space flight. Microgravity Q 1992;2(2):89–102.

16. Booth FW. Terrestrial applications of bone and muscle research in microgravity. Adv Space Res 1994;14(8):373–6.

17. Kim YJ, Bonassar LJ, Grodzinsky AJ. The role of cartilage streaming potential, fluid flow and pressure in the stimulation of chondrocyte biosynthesis during dynamic compression. J Biomech 1995;28(9):1055–66.

18. Waldman SD, Spiteri CG, Grynpas MD, et al. Long-term intermittent shear deformation improves the quality of cartilaginous tissue formed in vitro. J Orthop Res 2003;21(4):590–6.

19. Carter DR, Beaupre GS, Wong M, et al. The mechanobiology of articular cartilage development and degeneration. Clin Orthop Relat Res 2004;(Suppl 427): S69–77.

20. Carter DR, Wong M. Mechanical stresses and endochondral ossification in the chondroepiphysis. J Orthop Res 1988;6(1):148–54.

21. Carter DR, Wong M. The role of mechanical loading histories in the development of diarthrodial joints. J Orthop Res 1988;6(6):804–16.

22. Wong M, Carter DR. Articular cartilage functional histomorphology and mechanobiology: a research perspective. Bone 2003;33(1):1–13.

23. Sandor SM, Hart JA, Oakes BW. Case study: rehabilitation of a surgically repaired medial collateral knee ligament using a limited motion cast and isokinetic exercise*. J Orthop Sports Phys Ther 1986; 7(4):154–8.

24. Haapala J, Arokoski JP, Hyttinen MM, et al. Remobilization does not fully restore immobilization induced articular cartilage atrophy. Clin Orthop Relat Res 1999;(362):218–29.

25. Helminen HJ, Jurvelin J, Kuusela T, et al. Effects of immobilization for 6 weeks on rabbit knee articular surfaces as assessed by the semiquantitative stereomicroscopic method. Acta Anat (Basel) 1983;115(4): 327–35.

26. Jurvelin J, Kiviranta I, Tammi M, et al. Softening of canine articular cartilage after immobilization of the knee joint. Clin Orthop Relat Res 1986;(207): 246–52.

27. Paukkonen K, Helminen HJ, Tammi M, et al. Quantitative morphological and biochemical investigations on the effects of physical exercise and immobilization on the articular cartilage of young rabbits. Acta Biol Hung 1984;35(2–4):293–304.

28. Paukkonen K, Jurvelin J, Helminen HJ. Effects of immobilization on the articular cartilage in young rabbits. A quantitative light microscopic stereological study. Clin Orthop Relat Res 1986;(206):270–80.

29. Tammi M, Saamanen AM, Jauhiainen A, et al. Proteoglycan alterations in rabbit knee articular cartilage following physical exercise and immobilization. Connect Tissue Res 1983;11(1):45–55.

30. Kim HK, Kerr RG, Cruz TF, et al. Effects of continuous passive motion and immobilization on synovitis and cartilage degradation in antigen induced arthritis. J Rheumatol 1995;22(9):1714–21.

31. Salter RB. The biologic concept of continuous passive motion of synovial joints. The first 18 years

of basic research and its clinical application. Clin Orthop Relat Res 1989;(242):12–25.

32. Salter RB, Simmonds DF, Malcolm BW, et al. The biological effect of continuous passive motion on the healing of full-thickness defects in articular cartilage. An experimental investigation in the rabbit. J Bone Joint Surg Am 1980;62(8):1232–51.

33. Ghadially FN. Fine structure of the joint. In: Sokoloff L, editor. The Joints and Synovial Fluid. New York: Academic press; 1978. p. 105–76.

34. Ogata K, Whiteside LA, Lesker PA. Subchondral route for nutrition to articular cartilage in the rabbit. Measurement of diffusion with hydrogen gas in vivo. J Bone Joint Surg Am 1978;60(7):905–10.

35. Muir H. The chondrocyte, architect of cartilage. Biomechanics, structure, function and molecular biology of cartilage matrix macromolecules. Bioessays 1995;17(12):1039–48.

36. Poole CA, Flint MH, Beaumont BW. Chondrons in cartilage: ultrastructural analysis of the pericellular microenvironment in adult human articular cartilages. J Orthop Res 1987;5(4):509–22.

37. Szirmai JA, Larsson T. Structure of cartilage. Stockholm (Sweden): Nordiska Bokhandelns; 1969. p. 163–84.

38. Hing WA, Sherwin AF, Poole CA. The influence of the pericellular microenvironment on the chondrocyte response to osmotic challenge. Osteoarthr Cartil 2002;10(4):297–307.

39. Sherwin AF, Carter DH, Poole CA, et al. The distribution of type VI collagen in the developing tissues of the bovine femoral head. Histochem J 1999; 31(9):623–32.

40. Roth V, Mow VC. The intrinsic tensile behavior of the matrix of bovine articular cartilage and its variation with age. J Bone Joint Surg Am 1980;62(7):1102–17.

41. Hwang WS, Li B, Jin LH, et al. Collagen fibril structure of normal, aging, and osteoarthritic cartilage. J Pathol 1992;167(4):425–33.

42. Poole AR, Rizkalla G, Ionescu M, et al. Osteoarthritis in the human knee: a dynamic process of cartilage matrix degradation, synthesis and reorganization. Agents Actions Suppl 1993;39:3–13.

43. Venn M, Maroudas A. Chemical composition and swelling of normal and osteoarthrotic femoral head cartilage. I. Chemical composition. Ann Rheum Dis 1977;36(2):121–9.

44. Kuettner KE, Aydelotte MB, Thonar EJ. Articular cartilage matrix and structure: a minireview. J Rheumatol Suppl 1991;27:46–8.

45. Quintarelli G, Ippolito E, Roden L. Age-dependent changes on the state of aggregation of cartilage matrix. Lab Invest 1975;32(1):111–23.

46. Smith JW, Peters TJ, Serafini-Fracassini A. Observations on the distribution of the proteinpolysaccharide complex and collagen in bovine articular cartilage. J Cell Sci 1967;2(1):129–36.

47. Mathews MB. The interaction of collagen and acid mucopolysaccharides. A model for connective tissue. Biochem J 1965;96(3):710–6.

48. Hamerman D, Rosenberg LC, Schubert M. Diarthrodial joints revisited. J Bone Joint Surg Am 1970;52(4):725–74.

49. Durr J, Lammi P, Goodman SL, et al. Identification and immunolocalization of laminin in cartilage. Exp Cell Res 1996;222(1):225–33.

50. Hedbom E, Antonsson P, Hjerpe A, et al. Cartilage matrix proteins. An acidic oligomeric protein (COMP) detected only in cartilage. J Biol Chem 1992;267(9):6132–6.

51. Muller G, Michel A, Altenburg E. COMP (cartilage oligomeric matrix protein) is synthesized in ligament, tendon, meniscus, and articular cartilage. Connect Tissue Res 1998;39(4):233–44.

52. Guilak F, Alexopoulos LG, Upton ML, et al. The pericellular matrix as a transducer of biomechanical and biochemical signals in articular cartilage. Ann N Y Acad Sci 2006;1068:498–512.

53. Eyre DR. The collagens of articular cartilage. Semin Arthritis Rheum 1991;21(3 Suppl 2):2–11.

54. Eyre DR, Wu JJ. Collagen structure and cartilage matrix integrity. J Rheumatol Suppl 1995;43:82–5.

55. Eyre DR, Wu JJ, Apone S. A growing family of collagens in articular cartilage: identification of 5 genetically distinct types. J Rheumatol 1987; 14(Spec No):25–37.

56. Eyre DR, Wu JJ, Woods PE. The cartilage collagens: structural and metabolic studies. J Rheumatol Suppl 1991;27:49–51.

57. Mayne R. Cartilage collagens. What is their function, and are they involved in articular disease? Arthritis Rheum 1989;32(3):241–6.

58. Akizuki S, Mow VC, Muller F, et al. Tensile properties of human knee joint cartilage: I. Influence of ionic conditions, weight bearing, and fibrillation on the tensile modulus. J Orthop Res 1986;4(4): 379–92.

59. Cremer MA, Rosloniec EF, Kang AH. The cartilage collagens: a review of their structure, organization, and role in the pathogenesis of experimental arthritis in animals and in human rheumatic disease. J Mol Med (Berl) 1998; 76(3–4):275–88.

60. Mendler M, Eich-Bender SG, Vaughan L, et al. Cartilage contains mixed fibrils of collagen types II, IX, and XI. J Cell Biol 1989;108(1):191–7.

61. Olsen BR. Collagen IX. Int J Biochem Cell Biol 1997;29(4):555–8.

62. Wu JJ, Eyre DR. Cartilage type IX collagen is cross-linked by hydroxypyridinium residues. Biochem Biophys Res Commun 1984;123(3):1033–9.

63. Wu JJ, Eyre DR. Covalent interactions of type IX collagen in cartilage. Connect Tissue Res 1989; 20(1–4):241–6.

64. Diab M, Wu JJ, Eyre DR. Collagen type IX from human cartilage: a structural profile of intermolecular cross-linking sites. Biochem J 1996;314(Pt 1): 327–32.

65. Hambach L, Neureiter D, Zeiler G, et al. Severe disturbance of the distribution and expression of type VI collagen chains in osteoarthritic articular cartilage. Arthritis Rheum 1998;41(6):986–96.

66. Soder S, Hambach L, Lissner R, et al. Ultrastructural localization of type VI collagen in normal adult and osteoarthritic human articular cartilage. Osteoarthr Cartil 2002;10(6):464–70.

67. Aigner T, Reichenberger E, Bertling W, et al. Type X collagen expression in osteoarthritic and rheumatoid articular cartilage. Virchows Arch B Cell Pathol Incl Mol Pathol 1993;63(4):205–11.

68. Gannon JM, Walker G, Fischer M, et al. Localization of type X collagen in canine growth plate and adult canine articular cartilage. J Orthop Res 1991;9(4):485–94.

69. Nerlich AG, Kirsch T, Wiest I, et al. Localization of collagen X in human fetal and juvenile articular cartilage and bone. Histochemistry 1992;98(5): 275–81.

70. von der Mark K, Kirsch T, Nerlich A, et al. Type X collagen synthesis in human osteoarthritic cartilage. Indication of chondrocyte hypertrophy. Arthritis Rheum 1992;35(7):806–11.

71. Takahashi M, Kushida K, Hoshino H, et al. Concentrations of pyridinoline and deoxypyridinoline in joint tissues from patients with osteoarthritis or rheumatoid arthritis. Ann Rheum Dis 1996;55(5): 324–7.

72. Takahashi M, Kushida K, Ohishi T, et al. Quantitative analysis of crosslinks pyridinoline and pentosidine in articular cartilage of patients with bone and joint disorders. Arthritis Rheum 1994;37(5):724–8.

73. Eleswarapu SV, Responte DJ, Athanasiou KA. Tensile properties, collagen content, and crosslinks in connective tissues of the immature knee joint. PLoS One 2011;6(10):e26178.

74. Eyre DR, Dickson IR, Van Ness K. Collagen crosslinking in human bone and articular cartilage. Age-related changes in the content of mature hydroxypyridinium residues. Biochem J 1988;252(2): 495–500.

75. Ratcliffe AM, Mow VC. Articular cartilage. In: Comper WD, editor. Extracellular Matrix, vol. 1. Amsterdam: Harwood Academic Publishers; 1996. p. 234–302.

76. Inerot S, Heinegard D, Audell L, et al. Articular-cartilage proteoglycans in aging and osteoarthritis. Biochem J 1978;169(1):143–56.

77. Hagg R, Bruckner P, Hedbom E. Cartilage fibrils of mammals are biochemically heterogeneous: differential distribution of decorin and collagen IX. J Cell Biol 1998;142(1):285–94.

78. Newton G, Weremowicz S, Morton CC, et al. Characterization of human and mouse cartilage oligomeric matrix protein. Genomics 1994;24(3):435–9.

79. Bianco P, Fisher LW, Young MF, et al. Expression and localization of the two small proteoglycans biglycan and decorin in developing human skeletal and non-skeletal tissues. J Histochem Cytochem 1990;38(11):1549–63.

80. Neame PJ, Choi HU, Rosenberg LC. The primary structure of the core protein of the small, leucine-rich proteoglycan (PG I) from bovine articular cartilage. J Biol Chem 1989;264(15):8653–61.

81. Poole AR, Rosenberg LC, Reiner A, et al. Contents and distributions of the proteoglycans decorin and biglycan in normal and osteoarthritic human articular cartilage. J Orthop Res 1996;14(5):681–9.

82. Scott PG, Dodd CM, Pringle GA. Mapping the locations of the epitopes of five monoclonal antibodies to the core protein of dermatan sulfate proteoglycan II (decorin). J Biol Chem 1993;268(16): 11558–64.

83. Burton-Wurster N, Lust G. Fibronectin and water content of articular cartilage explants after partial depletion of proteoglycans. J Orthop Res 1986; 4(4):437–45.

84. Couchman JR, Austria MR, Woods A. Fibronectin-cell interactions. J Invest Dermatol 1990;94(Suppl 6): 7S–14S.

85. Piperno M, Reboul P, Hellio le Graverand MP, et al. Osteoarthritic cartilage fibrillation is associated with a decrease in chondrocyte adhesion to fibronectin. Osteoarthr Cartil 1998;6(6):393–9.

86. Paulsson M, Heinegard D. Noncollagenous cartilage proteins current status of an emerging research field. Coll Relat Res 1984;4(3):219–29.

87. Tondravi MM, Winterbottom N, Haudenschild DR, et al. Cartilage matrix protein binds to collagen and plays a role in collagen fibrillogenesis. Prog Clin Biol Res 1993;383B:515–22.

88. Mollenhauer J, Bee JA, Lizarbe MA, et al. Role of anchorin CII, a 31,000-mol-wt membrane protein, in the interaction of chondrocytes with type II collagen. J Cell Biol 1984;98(4):1572–9.

89. Mollenhauer J, Mok MT, King KB, et al. Expression of anchorin CII (cartilage annexin V) in human young, normal adult, and osteoarthritic cartilage. J Histochem Cytochem 1999;47(2):209–20.

90. Carsons S, Horn VJ. Chondronectin in human synovial fluid. Ann Rheum Dis 1988;47(10):797–800.

91. Kahn A, Taitz AD, Pottenger LA, et al. Effect of link protein and free hyaluronic acid binding region on spacing of proteoglycans in aggregates. J Orthop Res 1994;12(5):612–20.

92. Broom ND, Poole CA. A functional-morphological study of the tidemark region of articular cartilage maintained in a non-viable physiological condition. J Anat 1982;135(Pt 1):65–82.

93. Havelka S, Horn V, Spohrova D, et al. The calcified-noncalcified cartilage interface: the tidemark. Acta Biol Hung 1984;35(2–4):271–9.

94. Benninghof A. Form und bau der gelenkknorpel in ihren beziehungen zur function. II. Der aufbau des gelenkknorpels in seinen beziehungen zur function. Z Zellforsch Mikrosk Anat 1925;2:783–862.

95. Hunziker EB. Articular cartilage structure in humans and experimental animals. In: Kuettner KE, Schleyerbach R, Peyron JG, et al, editors. Articular cartilage and osteoarthritis. New York: Raven Press Ltd; 1992. p. 183–99.

96. Mitrovic D, Quintero M, Stankovic A, et al. Cell density of adult human femoral condylar articular cartilage. Joints with normal and fibrillated surfaces. Lab Invest 1983;49(3):309–16.

97. Puig-Rosado A. Articular chondrogenesis. An experimental study in immature rabbits. J Bone Joint Surg Br 1981;63(4):619–22.

98. Jadin KD, Bae WC, Schumacher BL, et al. Three-dimensional (3-D) imaging of chondrocytes in articular cartilage: growth-associated changes in cell organization. Biomaterials 2007; 28(2):230–9.

99. Maroudas A, Muir H, Wingham J. The correlation of fixed negative charge with glycosaminoglycan content of human articular cartilage. Biochim Biophys Acta 1969;177(3):492–500.

100. Stockwell RA. Chondrocyte Metabolism. In: Harrison RJ, McMinn RMH, Treherne JE, editors. Biology of cartilage cells. Biological structure and function - Series 7. United Kingdom: Cambridge University Press; 1979. p. 81–123.

101. Muir H, Bullough P, Maroudas A. The distribution of collagen in human articular cartilage with some of its physiological implications. J Bone Joint Surg Br 1970;52(3):554–63.

102. Poole AC. Chondrons: the chondrocyte and its pericellular microenvironment. In: Kuettner KE, Schleyerbach R, Peyron JC, et al, editors. Articular Cartilage and Osteoarthritis. New York: Academic Press; 1992. p. 201–20.

103. Glant TT, Hadhazy C, Mikecz K, et al. Appearance and persistence of fibronectin in cartilage. Specific interaction of fibronectin with collagen type II. Histochemistry 1985;82(2):149–58.

104. Mason RM. Recent advances in the biochemistry of hyaluronic acid in cartilage. Prog Clin Biol Res 1981;54:87–112.

105. Miosge N, Flachsbart K, Goetz W, et al. Light and electron microscopical immunohistochemical localization of the small proteoglycan core proteins decorin and biglycan in human knee joint cartilage. Histochem J 1994;26(12):939–45.

106. Poole CA. Articular cartilage chondrons: form, function and failure. J Anat 1997;191(Pt 1):1–13.

107. Poole CA, Flint MH, Beaumont BW. Morphological and functional interrelationships of articular cartilage matrices. J Anat 1984;138(Pt 1):113–38.

108. Poole CA, Flint MH, Beaumont BW. Morphology of the pericellular capsule in articular cartilage revealed by hyaluronidase digestion. J Ultrastruct Res 1985;91(1):13–23.

109. Venn MF. Variation of chemical composition with age in human femoral head cartilage. Ann Rheum Dis 1978;37(2):168–74.

110. Broom ND, Flachsmann R. Physical indicators of cartilage health: the relevance of compliance, thickness, swelling and fibrillar texture. J Anat 2003;202(6):481–94.

111. Renstrom P. Sports traumatology today. A review of common current sports injury problems. Ann Chir Gynaecol 1991;80(2):81–93.

112. Stehling C, Lane NE, Nevitt MC, et al. Subjects with higher physical activity levels have more severe focal knee lesions diagnosed with 3T MRI: analysis of a non-symptomatic cohort of the osteoarthritis initiative. Osteoarthr Cartil 2010;18(6):776–86.

113. Wren TA, Beaupre GS, Carter DR. A model for loading-dependent growth, development, and adaptation of tendons and ligaments. J Biomech 1998;31(2):107–14.

114. Roos EM, Dahlberg L. Positive effects of moderate exercise on glycosaminoglycan content in knee cartilage: a four-month, randomized, controlled trial in patients at risk of osteoarthritis. Arthritis Rheum 2005;52(11):3507–14.

115. Foley S, Ding C, Cicuttini F, et al. Physical activity and knee structural change: a longitudinal study using MRI. Med Sci Sports Exerc 2007;39(3):426–34.

116. Hohmann E, Wortler K, Imhoff A. Osteoarthritis from long-distance running? Sportverletz Sportschaden 2005;19(2):89–93 [in German].

117. Gratzke C, Hudelmaier M, Hitzl W, et al. Knee cartilage morphologic characteristics and muscle status of professional weight lifters and sprinters: a magnetic resonance imaging study. Am J Sports Med 2007;35(8):1346–53.

118. Racunica TL, Teichtahl AJ, Wang Y, et al. Effect of physical activity on articular knee joint structures in community-based adults. Arthritis Rheum 2007; 57(7):1261–8.

119. Burt LA, Naughton GA, Greene DA, et al. Non-elite gymnastics participation is associated with greater bone strength, muscle size, and function in pre- and early pubertal girls. Osteoporos Int 2012; 23(4):1277–86.

120. Morris FL, Naughton GA, Gibbs JL, et al. Prospective ten-month exercise intervention in premenarcheal girls: positive effects on bone and lean mass. J Bone Miner Res 1997;12(9):1453–62.

121. Quiterio AL, Silva AM, Minderico CS, et al. Total body water measurements in adolescent athletes:

a comparison of six field methods with deuterium dilution. J Strength Cond Res 2009;23(4):1225–37.

122. Rogers RS, Hinton PS. Bone loading during young adulthood predicts bone mineral density in physically active, middle-aged men. Phys Sportsmed 2010;38(2):146–55.

123. Roemhildt ML, Beynnon BD, Gardner-Morse M, et al. Changes induced by chronic in vivo load alteration in the tibiofemoral joint of mature rabbits. J Orthop Res 2012. [Epub ahead of print]. DOI: 10.1002/jor.22087.

124. Lacourt M, Gao C, Li A, et al. Relationship between cartilage and subchondral bone lesions in repetitive impact trauma-induced equine osteoarthritis. Osteoarthr Cartil 2012. [Epub ahead of print].

125. Firth EC, Rogers CW, Perkins NR, et al. Musculoskeletal responses of 2-year-old thoroughbred horses to early training. 1. Study design, and clinical, nutritional, radiological and histological observations. N Z Vet J 2004;52(5):261–71.

126. Taes YE, Lapauw B, Vanbillemont G, et al. Fat mass is negatively associated with cortical bone size in young healthy male siblings. J Clin Endocrinol Metab 2009;94(7):2325–31.

127. Messier SP, Gutekunst DJ, Davis C, et al. Weight loss reduces knee-joint loads in overweight and obese older adults with knee osteoarthritis. Arthritis Rheum 2005;52(7):2026–32.

128. Luke AC, Stehling C, Stahl R, et al. High-field magnetic resonance imaging assessment of articular cartilage before and after marathon running: does long-distance running lead to cartilage damage? Am J Sports Med 2010;38(11):2273–80.

129. Hovis KK, Stehling C, Souza RB, et al. Physical activity is associated with magnetic resonance imaging-based knee cartilage T2 measurements in asymptomatic subjects with and those without osteoarthritis risk factors. Arthritis Rheum 2011;63(8):2248–56.

130. Pauwels F. Biomechanics of the locomotion apparatus. Berlin: Springer; 1980.

131. Carter DR, Wong M, Orr TE. Musculoskeletal ontogeny, phylogeny, and functional adaptation. J Biomech 1991;24(Suppl 1):3–16.

132. Huiskes R, Ruimerman R, van Lenthe GH, et al. Effects of mechanical forces on maintenance and adaptation of form in trabecular bone. Nature 2000; 405(6787):704–6.

133. Ateshian GA, Lai WM, Zhu WB, et al. An asymptotic solution for the contact of two biphasic cartilage layers. J Biomech 1994;27(11):1347–60.

134. Mow VC, Gu WY, Chen FH. Structure and function of articular cartilage and meniscus. In: Mow VC, Huiskes R, editors. Basic orthopaedic biomechanics and mechanobiology. 3rd edition. Philadelphia: Lippincott, Williams & Wilkins; 2003. p. 181–258.

135. Krishnan R, Park S, Eckstein F, et al. Inhomogeneous cartilage properties enhance superficial interstitial fluid support and frictional properties, but do not provide a homogeneous state of stress. J Biomech Eng 2003;125(5):569–77.

136. Jones G, Ding C, Glisson M, et al. Knee articular cartilage development in children: a longitudinal study of the effect of sex, growth, body composition, and physical activity. Pediatric Research 2003;54(2):230–6.

137. Jones G, Glisson M, Hynes K, et al. Sex and site differences in cartilage development: a possible explanation for variations in knee osteoarthritis in later life. Arthritis and Rheumatism 2000;43(11):2543–9.

138. Firth EC. The response of bone, articular cartilage and tendon to exercise in the horse. Journal of Anatomy 2006;208(4):513–26.

139. Daly RM. The effect of exercise on bone mass and structural geometry during growth. Medicine and Sport Science 2007;51:33–49.

140. Falk B, Galili Y, Zigel L, et al. A cumulative effect of physical training on bone strength in males. International Journal of Sports Medicine 2007;28(6): 449–55.

141. Roos EM, Dahlberg L. [Physical activity as medication against arthrosis–training has a positive effect on the cartilage]. Lakartidningen 2004;101(25): 2178–81.

142. Maffulli N, King JB. Effects of physical activity on some components of the skeletal system. Sports Medicine. (Auckland, NZ) 1992;13(6):393–407.

Imaging of Osteochondritis Dissecans

Aiden Moktassi, MD, FRCPC[a],*, Charles A. Popkin, MD[b],
Lawrence M. White, MD, FRCPC[a],
M. Lucas Murnaghan, MD, MEd, FRCSC[c]

KEYWORDS

- Osteochondritis dissecans • MRI • Articular cartilage

Osteochondritis dissecans (OCD) is an uncommon, localized process that affects the subchondral bone and can result in delamination and destabilization of the overlying articular cartilage.[1,2] This condition has been seen with increased frequency as children of younger age are participating in more competitive sports.[3] The incidence of OCD has been estimated to be between 0.02% and 0.03% by radiography, and as high as 1.2% by arthroscopy.[4,5] Prevalence of this condition ranges between 15 and 29 per 100,000,[6] with an increased male predominance of 2:1.[6] The knee is the most common location for OCD and the condition is bilateral in 15% to 30% of cases.[7] The classic location for OCD in the knee is the posterolateral aspect of the medial femoral condyle (69%).[8] Less common locations include the lateral femoral condyle (15%), patella (5%), and femoral trochlea (1%). Although not the focus of this discussion, other joints that can be affected include the ankle, elbow, hip, and wrist.

The etymology of the term osteochondritis dissecans is worthy of discussion. The *itis* suffix of osteochondritis denotes the previously understood cause of inflammation of the osteochondral joint surface. Dissecans is derived from Latin and means to separate. Franz Konig introduced the term osteochondritis dissecans in 1888, although it was originally described by Paget some years earlier.[9]

Although many researchers have attempted to determine the cause of OCD, there remains considerable debate and no clear consensus. Hereditary, traumatic, and vascular causes have been proposed, with conflicting evidence supporting each.[10–12] The ultimate cause of OCD lesions is unknown at this time, but is likely multifactorial, with mechanical causal factors being most important.

CLINICAL PRESENTATION

Early presentation of OCD often consists of vague pain in and around the knee. The pain is worse with activity and can be associated with an antalgic, externally rotated gait. If the lesion is unstable, mechanical symptoms may be present. On evaluation of the knee, the clinician may notice atrophy of the quadriceps and pain with range of motion.[3] The Wilson test is a special provocative test that has been described with attempts to impinge the tibial spine on the OCD lesion.[13] This test has more recently been shown to lack a satisfactory sensitivity and specificity, but can be used as

The authors have nothing to disclose.
[a] Department of Medical Imaging, Mount Sinai Hospital, University of Toronto, 600 University Avenue, Toronto, Ontario M5G 1X5, Canada
[b] Division of Orthopaedic Surgery, The Hospital for Sick Children, University of Toronto, 555 University Avenue, Toronto, Ontario M5G 1X8, Canada
[c] Division of Orthopaedic Surgery, Department of Surgery, The Hospital for Sick Children, University of Toronto, 555 University Avenue, Toronto, Ontario M5G 1X8, Canada
* Corresponding author.
E-mail address: aiden.moktassi@gmail.com

Orthop Clin N Am 43 (2012) 201–211
doi:10.1016/j.ocl.2012.01.001

a test after treatment to assess for clinical healing.[14]

IMAGING WORK-UP

Because of the nonspecific nature of the clinical signs and symptoms of OCD, imaging plays a central role in the diagnosis and prognosis of this disease. The role of the different imaging modalities has evolved with time. Imaging modalities used for assessment of OCD include conventional radiography, nuclear medicine, computed tomography (CT), CT arthrography, magnetic resonance imaging (MRI), and magnetic resonance (MR) arthrography.

Conventional Radiography

Conventional radiographs allow determination of the size and location of the lesion as well as assessment of the skeletal maturity of the patient. Initial radiographic evaluation of patients with suspected OCD should include anterior-posterior (AP), lateral, tunnel, and skyline views. The tunnel view provides improved visualization of the posterior aspect of the femoral condyle as it is brought into view with knee flexion (**Fig. 1**). The skyline view allows for visualization of the femoral trochlea, an uncommon but problematic location for OCD lesions. Imaging of the contralateral knee should be considered if symptoms warrant it.

Characteristic radiographic findings include a well-circumscribed area of subchondral bone separated by a crescent-shaped radiolucent outline of the fragment. Although the radiographic examination can establish the diagnosis of OCD correctly, it is not adequate for prognostic and therapeutic decisions. This limitation is often caused by discrepancies between surgical and radiographic manifestations of the disease.[5] Discrepancies include underestimation of fragment size, or fragments that appear radiographically separated can be covered by normal cartilage at surgery, and vice versa (**Fig. 2**).[5,15] In general, conventional radiographs are poor at establishing the stability and size of the lesion and are unable to assess the status of the overlying cartilage.[16,17] In addition, radiographs may not always show OCD lesions consistently or definitively.[17]

Bone Scan

Nuclear medicine technetium-99m methylene diphosphonate (MDP) bone scans have been investigated and used as a potential dynamic study to evaluate the healing potential of OCD defects.[18–20] In comparison with radiography, scintigraphy has superior sensitivity to changes in the stability of OCD lesions.[18] This technique was initially thought useful in determining the need for operative intervention for lesions that show increased activity on bone scan despite conservative treatment. Another proposed advantage of scintigraphy is its ability to differentiate anomalies of ossification versus true OCD, with ossification anomalies having minimal, if any, increased radiotracer uptake.

With radionuclide scanning, findings between stable and unstable fragments overlap. Bone scintigraphy also provides no anatomic information on articular surface deformity. Hence, although bone scintigraphy can serve to localize a lesion to a specific joint, it often offers little specificity in

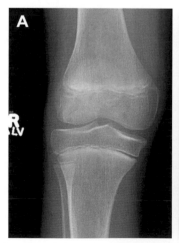 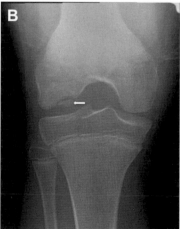

Fig. 1. A 14-year-old male patient with an OCD lesion on the lateral femoral condyle. (*A*) The abnormality of the articular surface is difficult to visualize on this view. The tunnel view (*B*) brings the posterior condyles into profile and clearly shows the lesion (*arrow*).

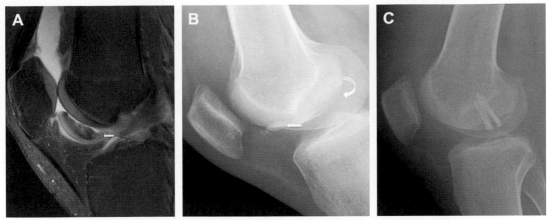

Fig. 2. Large partially ossified osteochondral fragment. (*A*) Sagittal 1.5-T (T) fast spin echo (FSE) T2-weighted MR image and (*B*) lateral radiograph shows the underestimation of the size of the mostly nonossified displaced osteochondral fragment situated anterior to the femoral trochlea (*arrow*). Large osteochondral defect at the lateral femoral condyle is also noted (*curved arrow*). (*C*) Postoperative lateral radiograph following rigid fixation of displaced osteochondral fragment with multiple headless screws.

distinguishing OCD lesions from other joint abnormalities. Bone scintigraphy has not been shown to provide reliable information about an OCD lesion's stability; as such, it has limited usefulness in differentiating surgical versus nonsurgical lesions.[19] In addition, bone scintigraphy requires exposure to ionizing radiation, can be time consuming, and requires an intravenous injection.

CT

CT offers excellent anatomic delineation of mineralized/ossified structures within the knee joint. However, conventional CT is poor at assessing articular cartilage and other noncalcified aspects of a joint. As such, conventional CT is limited in providing diagnostic information regarding OCD lesion stability or healing potential.

In contrast with conventional CT, CT arthrography has been used for cartilage imaging,[21] providing reliable information regarding the integrity of articular cartilage overlying an OCD lesion. CT arthrography consists of thin-slice CT evaluation following intra-articular administration of iodinated contrast. The introduction of spiral CT has provided the additional ability to obtain thin, overlapping CT sections with excellent secondary sagittal and coronal reformations. This evolution has resulted in a resurgence of CT arthrography for the assessment of intra-articular lesions, including OCD lesions.[22,23] However, given the young demographics of the typical OCD patient, the ionizing radiation associated with CT scanning has tempered widespread adoption.

MRI

MRI has been shown to be an ideal diagnostic technique for evaluation of OCD lesions because of its noninvasive nature, absence of ionizing radiation, excellent anatomic detail, and soft tissue contrast allowing cartilage visualization.

MRI has been shown to be diagnostically valuable in the differentiation of variations in ossification from true OCD lesions.[24] Ossification variability is typically seen as irregularity in the far-posterior condyles without intercondylar extension, and without associated edema (**Fig. 3**).[24] In contrast, true OCD lesions on MRI are seen as defects in the posterior femoral condyles with intercondylar extension and significant edema.

MRI is now commonly used to evaluate and confirm the presence of an OCD lesion but, more importantly, to assess stability of OCD lesions of the knee. Stability is the most important prognostic factor for determining the likelihood of an OCD lesion healing with nonoperative therapy.[3,25–28]

Multiple studies have described the MRI findings in patients with stable and unstable OCD lesions.[29–35] There are 4 widely used MRI criteria for OCD instability that were described by De Smet and colleagues (**Fig. 4**).[32,33] These MRI criteria include (1) a rim of high signal intensity surrounding an OCD lesion on T2-weighted images (hereafter referred to as high T2 signal intensity), (2) cysts surrounding an OCD lesion, (3) a fracture line of high T2 signal intensity extending through the articular cartilage overlying an OCD lesion, and (4) a fluid-filled osteochondral defect.

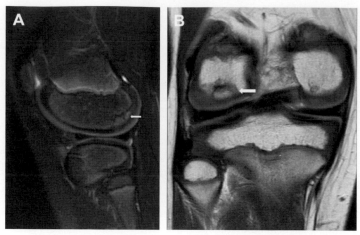

Fig. 3. A 12-year-old boy with ossification defect at the lateral femoral condyle. (*A*) Sagittal 1.5-T T2-weighted FSE MR image shows an ill-defined osteochondral lesion (*arrow*) in the posterior third of the lateral femoral condyle. No significant edema is noted. (*B*) Coronal intermediate-weighted fast spin-echo MR image shows a triangular-shaped ossification defect (*arrow*) of the central third of the lateral femoral condyle without inter-condylar extension.

Despite the popularity of these criteria, there is no apparent consensus in the literature regarding the most appropriate MRI criteria for defining OCD instability. The widespread difference of opinion may relate to a lack of distinction between the juvenile and adult forms OCD and the potentially different imaging features of stability/instability seen between juvenile and adult forms of the disease.

Recently, Kijowski and colleagues[36] proposed revised criteria for OCD instability based on skeletal maturity of the patient. In a study of 32 skeletally immature patients using arthroscopy as the reference standard, Kijowski and colleagues[36] found that the presence of T2 signal intensity rim or cysts surrounding an OCD lesion may be a sign of instability only in adults. In their cohort of juvenile patients, a rim of high T2 signal intensity surrounding an OCD lesion indicated instability only if it had the same signal intensity as adjacent joint fluid, was surrounded by a second outer rim of low T2 signal intensity (**Figs. 5** and **6**), or was accompanied by multiple breaks in the subchondral bone plate. Cysts surrounding a juvenile OCD lesion indicated instability only if they were multiple or large (>5 mm) in size.

The De Smet criteria[32,33] initially revealed a sensitivity and specificity of 92% and 90% respectively for differentiating unstable lesions from stable lesions.[30] However, subsequent

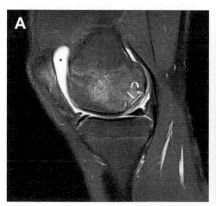
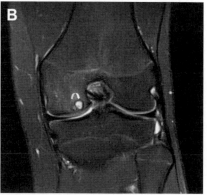

Fig. 4. A 21-year-old man with an unstable adult OCD lesion of the lateral femoral condyle. (*A*) Sagittal and (*B*) coronal 1.5-T FSE T2-weighted MR findings of a rim of high signal intensity (*straight arrow*) and cystic area (*curved arrow*) beneath the fragment. The presence of a joint effusion is also noted (*asterisk*).

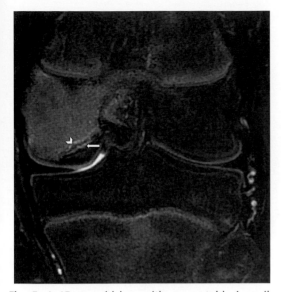

Fig. 5. A 15-year-old boy with an unstable juvenile OCD lesion of medial femoral condyle. Coronal 1.5-T fat-suppressed T2-weighted FSE MR image of an OCD lesion surrounded by an inner rim of high T2 signal intensity (*arrow*) and a second outer rim of low T2 signal intensity (*arrowhead*). There is also extensive bone marrow edema surrounding the lesion.

studies using the revised criteria of Kijowski and colleagues[36] showed sensitivities and specificities approaching 100%.

Some investigators have also recommended using direct MR arthrography for evaluating patients with OCD, looking for signs of instability and differentiation of partial versus complete separation of fragments indicated by contrast subsiding the OCD fragment (**Fig. 7**).[9,37,38] Direct MR arthrography also provides advantages of distention, increased intra-articular pressure from the fluid volume, and increased signal/noise ratio on T1-weighted imaging. However, these advantages come at the cost of converting a noninvasive examination (conventional MRI) to an invasive procedure, and there are the potential complications inherent to intra-articular injection of contrast material.[39]

MRI Sequences/Protocol

An ideal MRI protocol for accurate assessment of OCD lesions and OCD repair should provide accurate assessment of cartilage thickness, signal changes within cartilage, the cartilage and bone interface, and the subchondral bone. It should also provide valuable information about articular cartilage repair tissue after surgery.

There are multiple existing and developing MRI pulse sequences that are valuable in assessment of osteochondral lesions. Two classes of pulse sequence acquisition have been most widely used in this regard: intermediate and T2-weighted fast spin echo (FSE) techniques, and three-dimensional (3D) spoiled gradient echo (SPGR) or fast low-angle shot (FLASH) sequences.

Fat-suppressed 3D SPGR and FLASH acquisitions provide high-resolution images with high contrast between the bright cartilage and dark fluid, bone, fat, and muscle. In these sequences, cartilage abnormalities are seen as morphologic abnormalities of contour. Potential limitations of such sequences include their long acquisition

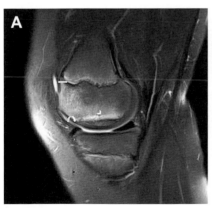
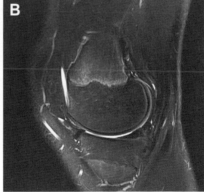

Fig. 6. (*A*) Sagittal 1.5-T T2-weighted FSE MR image of knee in a 12-year-old girl with a stable juvenile OCD lesion of the medial femoral condyle. The OCD lesion is surrounded by a rim of high T2 signal intensity (*arrowhead*) that has lower signal intensity than adjacent joint fluid (*arrow*). There is no disruption of the subchondral bone plate (low signal intensity) at the edges of OCD lesion (*curved arrow*). No cysts larger then 5 mm are noted. (*B*) Two-year follow-up sagittal 1.5-T T2-weighted FSE MR image shows interval healing with no residual OCD lesion identified.

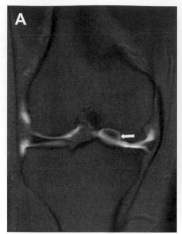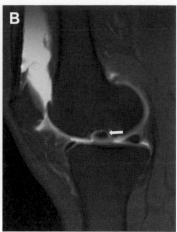

Fig. 7. MR arthrogram of an unstable adult OCD lesion of the medial femoral condyle. (*A*) Coronal and (*B*) sagittal T1-weighted fat saturation FSE images following intra-articular administration of gadolinium show a rim of contrast outlining an unstable medial femoral condyle OCD lesion (*arrows*).

times as well as their susceptibility to metal artifacts, which may be an important consideration after surgery.

Intermediate-weighted and T2-weighted FSE acquisitions provide high-resolution, high-contrast imaging of articular cartilage in a short acquisition time. Intermediate-weighted FSE imaging combines T2 weighting and relative fatty marrow signal preservation to generate images with bright joint fluid and subcortical bone marrow. This process results in an arthrogramlike effect and highlights the usually low-intermediate signal cartilage.[40] The addition of fat saturation to FSE techniques can help in the evaluation of articular cartilage by optimizing the dynamic range of the images. FSE imaging also allows diagnostic evaluation of other intra-articular structures, including subchondral bone.[40,41] Fluid-sensitive (T2) sequences should be obtained in all 3 standard planes. For example, OCD involving the trochlear sulcus is best evaluated on axial and sagittal images.[42]

MRI Higher Field Imaging and Advanced Techniques

MRI at 3.0 T has the potential advantage of imaging with higher spatial resolution at similar imaging acquisition times, compared with 1.5-T imaging.[43,44] This higher resolution may in turn improve diagnostic accuracy. These higher field strength scanners are increasingly available in clinical practice; however, randomized controlled trials are necessary to evaluate the diagnostic efficacy of this new technology.

Emerging MRI sequences have shown great potential for the physiologic assessment of cartilage repair tissue. The main quantitative

sequences are T2 mapping and delayed gadolinium contrast-enhanced MRI of cartilage (dGEMRIC). Quantitative T2 mapping has been correlated with type II collagen matrix organization within normal hyaline articular cartilage. The dGEMRIC imaging technique, which displays the distribution of negatively charged gadolinium-based MRI contrast material (gadopentetate dimeglumine) within cartilage, has been validated as an accurate marker of cartilage tissue glycosaminoglycan (GAG) concentration.[45] These techniques have been investigated as potential tools to characterize the histologic and biochemical composition and temporal maturation of repair tissue following osteochondral repair procedures. However, the clinical usefulness of these quantitative techniques remains uncertain.

TREATMENT OF OCD

Important factors to consider in the treatment of OCD include the skeletal maturity of the patient as well as the lesion's size, location, and stability. Nonoperative treatment is an appropriate initial treatment in a stable lesion in a juvenile patient. A variety of nonoperative approaches exist, including activity modification, cast immobilization, and brace treatment.

The success of nonoperative treatment of stable OCD lesions ranges from 50% to 66%.[25,46] In addition to failure of nonoperative management, other operative indications include stable lesions with physeal closure within 6 months, unstable/hinged lesions, detached lesions (loose bodies), and full-thickness loss of overlying articular cartilage identified by MRI.

The primary goal of surgical management of OCD should be to preserve native articular cartilage congruity whenever possible. Stable lesions that have failed nonoperative treatment are best treated with arthroscopic drilling, which can take the form of transarticular or retroarticular drilling. The purpose of the drilling is to create vascular channels to stimulate revascularization and promote healing of the lesion (marrow stimulation).[3] Excellent results are reported using both drilling techniques and there is no consensus as to which method is superior.[25,47–49]

For OCD lesions that are unstable, stabilization of the lesion should be the primary goal. Fibrous tissue may need to be debrided and, in some situations, bone grafting is required. A variety of internal fixation devices have been described, including bone pegs, bioabsorbable darts/nails/screws, and metal screws (**Fig. 8**). Fixation can be done arthroscopically or, if necessary, with use of an arthrotomy to gain necessary access. Although there have been encouraging results using internal fixation when the lesion is salvageable, this procedure is difficult. Loosening, failures of hardware, loose bodies, and hemarthrosis are reported complications of internal fixation for OCD lesions.

If the OCD lesion is not repairable, the surgeon must turn to salvage procedures. Options available in this situation include microfracture to help promote filling of the defect with pluripotent cells,[50] autologous chondrocyte implantation, osteochondral autograft (**Fig. 9**), and allograft.[3]

IMAGING TO ASSESS HEALING

Imaging plays an important role following treatment to determine the success of the surgical intervention by assessing healing, confirming articular cartilage congruity, and excluding surgical complications. Similar findings are assessed in the setting of both primary repair and salvage procedures.

With its superb soft tissue contrast, MRI is the ideal modality in the assessment of osteochondral repair. Posttreatment MRI evaluation should assess signal within the in-situ fragment or graft and adjacent bone marrow, osteochondral integration (bone and cartilage integration), and cartilage surface contour.[51,52]

Caution is needed in the interpretation of early postoperative MRI studies. A degree of edema can often be seen in the OCD fragment/graft during the initial postoperative period (first 12

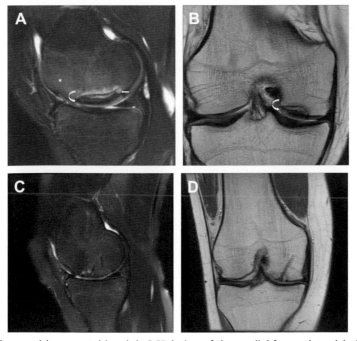

Fig. 8. A 21-year-old man with an unstable adult OCD lesion of the medial femoral condyle (*A*) Sagittal 1.5-T T2-weighted and (*B*) coronal intermediate-weighted FSE MR images show a large unstable adult OCD lesion of the medial femoral condyle with high T2 signal rim (*arrow*), cartilage cleft (*curved arrow*), and bone marrow edema (*asterisk*). (*C*) Sagittal T2-weighted and (*D*) coronal intermediate-weighted images acquired 18 months after arthroscopic bone grafting and fixation with multiple bioabsorbable screws show healing of the OCD lesion.

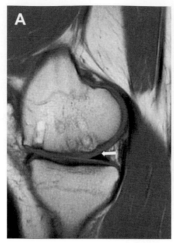
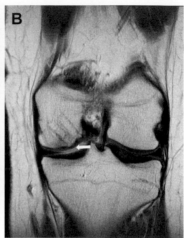

Fig. 9. A 28-year-old woman with unstable adult OCD treated with osteochondral autografting. (*A*) Sagittal and (*B*) coronal intermediate-weighted FSE images acquired 2 years following treatment show good integration of osteochondral plugs into the medial femoral condyle, with satisfactory articular cartilage congruency (*arrows*).

months). During the subsequent 12 months, signal intensity should return to normal.[52] Subchondral bone marrow edema seems to follow a similar pattern.[52–56]

The main focus of treatment is the congruity of the joint surface and the main criterion of technical success. Gaps or clefts at the integration zone of the graft or OCD fragment should be evaluated for. These clefts have the potential to progress to separation of the fragment or graft from the underlying femur.[57] A rim of fluid between the base of the repaired fragment or graft likely indicates an unstable repair.[57] Postoperative surface congruity improves over time with fibrocartilaginous tissue formation.[51]

In terms of microfracture treatment of OCD lesions, the MR appearance is often variable and changes over time. At first, the reparative tissue may be diminutive and indistinct, but, by 1 to 2 years, it often has filled the defect. MRI has been shown to be highly accurate, with correlation with lesion fill of up 100%.[58,59] There is also emerging evidence that the degree of defect fill on MRI may correlate with clinical outcome.[33]

Overall, persistent or increasing subchondral edema and incomplete filling of the defect are indicators of treatment failure.[57] Cyst formation or persistent edema at the subchondral bone are poor prognostic indicators and are associated with failure of bone integration.[55] Other complications assessed by MRI include fixation hardware complications (including fracture or malposition; **Figs. 10** and **11**), fragment/graft loosening or migration/displacement, cartilage-cartilage interface incongruence, gaps between the native

cartilage and OCD fragment/graft, autologous chondrocyte implantation graft hypertrophy, and OCD fragment/graft necrosis.[52] The presence of adhesions and joint effusion can also be evaluated.

Postoperative imaging follow-up is essential in the evaluation of healing. Initial short-term follow-up imaging (3–6 months) allows assessment of the integration of repair tissue. Subsequent long-term follow-up imaging allows an evaluation of the maturation of the OCD graft and identification of any complications. Although some investigators have judged MR arthrography to be superior to

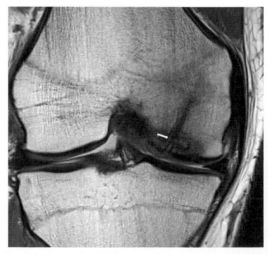

Fig. 10. Coronal 1.5-T intermediate-weighted FSE MR image acquired 6 months following OCD fixation shows fractured bioabsorbable screw (*arrow*).

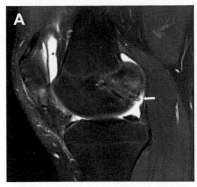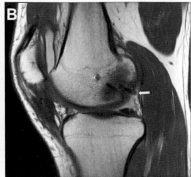

Fig. 11. (*A*) Sagittal 1.5-T T2-weighted fast spin-echo and (*B*) sagittal intermediate-weighted FSE MR images show proud placement of fixation screws following attempted OCD lesion rigid fixation (*arrow*). Note reactive effusion (*asterisk*).

conventional MRI,[57,60] others have reported the effective evaluation of repair tissue without the use of contrast agents.[58,61]

SUMMARY

Osteochondritis dissecans is a disorder involving the separation of a fragment of cartilage and bone from the joint surface. Given the nonspecific presentation of OCD, imaging plays a central role in the assessment of OCD. MRI has become the modality of choice for OCD with its clear superiority compared with plain radiography and bone scintigraphy. Although the definitive determination of instability can be challenging, cartilage-tailored sequences have improved diagnostic accuracy and subsequent clinical decision making. The distinction between juvenile and adult OCD lesions of the knee is important because these lesions have different MRI criteria for instability. Imaging also plays an important role in evaluating healing of OCD and articular congruity following surgical and nonsurgical management. Recent advances in MRI techniques may further understanding of this disorder and, in turn, improve its treatment and outcomes.

REFERENCES

1. Heywood CS, Benke MT, Brindle K, et al. Correlation of magnetic resonance imaging to arthroscopic findings of stability in juvenile osteochondritis dissecans. Arthroscopy 2011;27(2):194–9.
2. Crawford DC, Safran MR. Osteochondritis dissecans of the knee. J Am Acad Orthop Surg 2006; 14(2):90–100.
3. Kocher MS, Tucker R, Ganley TJ, et al. Management of osteochondritis dissecans of the knee: current concepts review. Am J Sports Med 2006;34(7): 1181–91.
4. Linden B. The incidence of osteochondritis dissecans in the condyles of the femur. Acta Orthop Scand 1976;47(6):664–7.
5. Bradley J, Dandy DJ. Osteochondritis dissecans and other lesions of the femoral condyles. J Bone Joint Surg Br 1989;71(3):518–22.
6. Hughston JC, Hergenroeder PT, Courtenay BG. Osteochondritis dissecans of the femoral condyles. J Bone Joint Surg Am 1984;66(9):1340–8.
7. Hefti F, Beguiristain J, Krauspe R, et al. Osteochondritis dissecans: a multicenter study of the European Pediatric Orthopedic Society. J Pediatr Orthop B 1999;8(4):231–45.
8. Aichroth P. Osteochondritis dissecans of the knee. A clinical survey. J Bone Joint Surg Br 1971;53(3):440–7.
9. Bohndorf K. Osteochondritis (osteochondrosis) dissecans: a review and new MRI classification. Eur Radiol 1998;8(1):103–12.
10. Mubarak SJ, Carroll NC. Familial osteochondritis dissecans of the knee. Clin Orthop Relat Res 1979;(140):131–6.
11. Petrie PW. Aetiology of osteochondritis dissecans. Failure to establish a familial background. J Bone Joint Surg Br 1977;59(3):366–7.
12. Ribbing S. Hereditare multiple Epiphysenstorungen und Osteochondrosis dissecans [Multiple hereditary epiphyseal disorders and osteochondrosis dissecans]. Acta Radiol 1951;36(5):397–404.
13. Wilson JN. A diagnostic sign in osteochondritis dissecans of the knee. J Bone Joint Surg Am 1967; 49(3):477–80.
14. Conrad JM, Stanitski CL. Osteochondritis dissecans: Wilson's sign revisited. Am J Sports Med 2003;31(5):777–8.
15. Pritsch M, Horoshovski H, Farine I. Arthroscopic treatment of osteochondral lesions of the talus. J Bone Joint Surg Am 1986;68(6):862–5.
16. Shanley DJ, Mulligan ME. Osteochondrosis dissecans of the glenoid. Skeletal Radiol 1990;19(6): 419–21.

17. Scott DJ Jr, Stevenson CA. Osteochondritis dissecans of the knee in adults. Clin Orthop Relat Res 1971;76:82–6.

18. Cahill BR, Berg BC. 99m-Technetium phosphate compound joint scintigraphy in the management of juvenile osteochondritis dissecans of the femoral condyles. Am J Sports Med 1983;11(5):329–35.

19. Bohndorf K. Injuries at the articulating surfaces of bone (chondral, osteochondral, subchondral fractures and osteochondrosis dissecans). Eur J Radiol 1996;22(1):22–9.

20. Vande Berg BC, Lecouvet FE, Poilvache P, et al. Spiral CT arthrography of the knee: technique and value in the assessment of internal derangement of the knee. Eur Radiol 2002;12(7):1800–10.

21. Reiser M, Karpf PM, Bernett P. Diagnosis of chondromalacia patellae using CT arthrography. Eur J Radiol 1982;2(3):181–6.

22. Vande Berg BC, Lecouvet FE, Poilvache P, et al. Assessment of knee cartilage in cadavers with dual-detector spiral CT arthrography and MR imaging. Radiology 2002;222(2):430–6.

23. Vande Berg BC, Lecouvet FE, Maldague B, et al. MR appearance of cartilage defects of the knee: preliminary results of a spiral CT arthrography-guided analysis. Eur Radiol 2004;14(2):208–14.

24. Jans LB, Jaremko JL, Ditchfield M, et al. MRI differentiates femoral condylar ossification evolution from osteochondritis dissecans. A new sign. Eur Radiol 2011;21(6):1170–9.

25. Cahill BR. Osteochondritis dissecans of the knee: treatment of juvenile and adult forms. J Am Acad Orthop Surg 1995;3(4):237–47.

26. Flynn JM, Kocher MS, Ganley TJ. Osteochondritis dissecans of the knee. J Pediatr Orthop 2004; 24(4):434–43.

27. Robertson W, Kelly BT, Green DW. Osteochondritis dissecans of the knee in children. Curr Opin Pediatr 2003;15(1):38–44.

28. Twyman RS, Desai K, Aichroth PM. Osteochondritis dissecans of the knee. A long-term study. J Bone Joint Surg Br 1991;73(3):461–4.

29. O'Connor MA, Palaniappan M, Khan N, et al. Osteochondritis dissecans of the knee in children. A comparison of MRI and arthroscopic findings. J Bone Joint Surg Br 2002;84(2):258–62.

30. Mesgarzadeh M, Sapega AA, Bonakdarpour A, et al. Osteochondritis dissecans: analysis of mechanical stability with radiography, scintigraphy, and MR imaging. Radiology 1987;165(3):775–80.

31. Nelson DW, DiPaola J, Colville M, et al. Osteochondritis dissecans of the talus and knee: prospective comparison of MR and arthroscopic classifications. J Comput Assist Tomogr 1990;14(5):804–8.

32. De Smet AA, Fisher DR, Graf BK, et al. Osteochondritis dissecans of the knee: value of MR imaging in determining lesion stability and the presence of articular cartilage defects. AJR Am J Roentgenol 1990;155(3):549–53.

33. De Smet AA, Ilahi OA, Graf BK. Reassessment of the MR criteria for stability of osteochondritis dissecans in the knee and ankle. Skeletal Radiol 1996;25(2): 159–63.

34. Yoshida S, Ikata T, Takai H, et al. Osteochondritis dissecans of the femoral condyle in the growth stage. Clin Orthop Relat Res 1998;(346):162–70.

35. Pill SG, Ganley TJ, Milam RA, et al. Role of magnetic resonance imaging and clinical criteria in predicting successful nonoperative treatment of osteochondritis dissecans in children. J Pediatr Orthop 2003; 23(1):102–8.

36. Kijowski R, Blankenbaker DG, Shinki K, et al. Juvenile versus adult osteochondritis dissecans of the knee: appropriate MR imaging criteria for instability. Radiology 2008;248(2):571–8.

37. Kramer J, Recht MP, Imhof H, et al. Postcontrast MR arthrography in assessment of cartilage lesions. J Comput Assist Tomogr 1994;18(2):218–24.

38. Kramer J, Stiglbauer R, Engel A, et al. MR contrast arthrography (MRA) in osteochondrosis dissecans. J Comput Assist Tomogr 1992;16(2):254–60.

39. Newberg AH, Munn CS, Robbins AH. Complications of arthrography. Radiology 1985;155(3):605–6.

40. McCauley TR, Recht MP, Disler DG. Clinical imaging of articular cartilage in the knee. Semin Musculoskelet Radiol 2001;5(4):293–304.

41. Recht MP, Goodwin DW, Winalski CS, et al. MRI of articular cartilage: revisiting current status and future directions. AJR Am J Roentgenol 2005; 185(4):899–914.

42. Boutin RD, Januario JA, Newberg AH, et al. MR imaging features of osteochondritis dissecans of the femoral sulcus. AJR Am J Roentgenol 2003; 180(3):641–5.

43. Gandhi RT, Kuo R, Crues JV 3rd. Technical considerations and potential advantages of musculoskeletal imaging at 3.0 Tesla. Semin Musculoskelet Radiol 2008;12(3):185–95.

44. Welsch GH, Mamisch TC, Hughes T, et al. Advanced morphological and biochemical magnetic resonance imaging of cartilage repair procedures in the knee joint at 3 Tesla. Semin Musculoskelet Radiol 2008;12(3):196–211.

45. Bashir A, Gray ML, Boutin RD, et al. Glycosaminoglycan in articular cartilage: in vivo assessment with delayed Gd(DTPA)(2-)-enhanced MR imaging. Radiology 1997;205(2):551–8.

46. Wall EJ, Vourazeris J, Myer GD, et al. The healing potential of stable juvenile osteochondritis dissecans knee lesions. J Bone Joint Surg Am 2008; 90(12):2655–64.

47. Donaldson LD, Wojtys EM. Extraarticular drilling for stable osteochondritis dissecans in the skeletally immature knee. J Pediatr Orthop 2008;28(8):831–5.

48. Adachi N, Deie M, Nakamae A, et al. Functional and radiographic outcome of stable juvenile osteochondritis dissecans of the knee treated with retroarticular drilling without bone grafting. Arthroscopy 2009; 25(2):145–52.

49. Kocher MS, Micheli LJ, Yaniv M, et al. Functional and radiographic outcome of juvenile osteochondritis dissecans of the knee treated with transarticular arthroscopic drilling. Am J Sports Med 2001;29(5): 562–6.

50. Steadman JR, Briggs KK, Rodrigo JJ, et al. Outcomes of microfracture for traumatic chondral defects of the knee: average 11-year follow-up. Arthroscopy 2003;19(5):477–84.

51. Trattnig S, Domayer S, Welsch GW, et al. MR imaging of cartilage and its repair in the knee— a review. Eur Radiol 2009;19(7):1582–94.

52. Domayer SE, Welsch GH, Dorotka R, et al. MRI monitoring of cartilage repair in the knee: a review. Semin Musculoskelet Radiol 2008;12(4):302–17.

53. Sanders TG, Mentzer KD, Miller MD, et al. Autogenous osteochondral "plug" transfer for the treatment of focal chondral defects: postoperative MR appearance with clinical correlation. Skeletal Radiol 2001; 30(10):570–8.

54. Sanders TG, Paruchuri NB, Zlatkin MB. MRI of osteochondral defects of the lateral femoral condyle: incidence and pattern of injury after transient lateral dislocation of the patella. AJR Am J Roentgenol 2006;187(5):1332–7.

55. Link TM, Mischung J, Wortler K, et al. Normal and pathological MR findings in osteochondral autografts with longitudinal follow-up. Eur Radiol 2006; 16(1):88–96.

56. Herber S, Runkel M, Pitton MB, et al. Indirect MR-arthrography in the follow up of autologous osteochondral transplantation. Rofo 2003;175(2):226–33 [in German].

57. Alparslan L, Winalski CS, Boutin RD, et al. Postoperative magnetic resonance imaging of articular cartilage repair. Semin Musculoskelet Radiol 2001;5(4): 345–63.

58. Mithoefer K, Williams RJ 3rd, Warren RF, et al. The microfracture technique for the treatment of articular cartilage lesions in the knee. A prospective cohort study. J Bone Joint Surg Am 2005;87(9): 1911–20.

59. Ramappa AJ, Gill TJ, Bradford CH, et al. Magnetic resonance imaging to assess knee cartilage repair tissue after microfracture of chondral defects. J Knee Surg 2007;20(3):228–34.

60. Ho YY, Stanley AJ, Hui JH, et al. Postoperative evaluation of the knee after autologous chondrocyte implantation: what radiologists need to know. Radiographics 2007;27(1):207–20 [discussion: 221–2].

61. Brown WE, Potter HG, Marx RG, et al. Magnetic resonance imaging appearance of cartilage repair in the knee. Clin Orthop Relat Res 2004;(422): 214–23.

Epidemiology, Pathogenesis, and Imaging of Arthritis in Children

Ricardo Restrepo, MD[a],*, Edward Y. Lee, MD, MPH[b]

KEYWORDS

- Juvenile idiopathic arthritis • Pathogenesis • Synovitis
- Imaging

Juvenile idiopathic arthritis (JIA) is a broad term that includes all forms of arthritis of unknown cause with onset before 16 years of age and that persist for at least 6 weeks in children and adolescents. A diagnosis of JIA is based mainly on clinical findings rather than on laboratory tests or imaging findings. Although the hallmark of all subtypes of JIA is synovial inflammation, the pathogenesis of each subtype differs. No imaging protocols have yet been established for JIA; however, a familiarity with imaging modalities and their indications proves helpful when attempting to answer specific questions to better define, classify, and treat patients with JIA.

EPIDEMIOLOGY

JIA is the most common chronic rheumatologic childhood disease, with an onset before 16 years of age and persisting for at least 6 weeks. It occurs in a worldwide distribution with regional variations thought to be due to differences in the distribution of HLA alleles and environmental factors.[1] Among developed nations, JIA has a yearly incidence rate of 2 to 20 cases per 100,000 population and a prevalence of 16 to 150 cases per 100,000 population.[2] In a comprehensive survey of data from 2002, the incidence of chronic arthritis of childhood ranged from 0.008 to 0.226 per 1000 children and the prevalence from 0.07 to 4.01 per 1000 children worldwide.[3] The true incidence of JIA is believed to vary widely, however, in part because it is composed of a heterogeneous group of arthritic conditions that are clinically diagnosed.[4] In a multiethnic cohort study by Saurenmann and colleagues,[4] European ancestry was shown an important predisposing factor for developing all types of JIA, in particular the oligoarticular and psoriatic subtypes, except the rheumatoid factor (RF)-positive polyarticular type. In this study, native North American children were also found at a higher risk of developing polyarticular disease than children of European descent.

CLASSIFICATION

JIA is a broad term that was developed by the International League of Associations for Rheumatology (ILAR) to group chronic arthritis in patients younger than 16 years of age for research purposes. This task force created relatively homogeneous, mutually exclusive categories of JIA based on clinical findings, replacing the terms, *juvenile chronic arthritis* and *juvenile rheumatoid arthritis*.[4–6] JIA encompasses a heterogeneous group of diseases classified into 7 subtypes according to age of onset, number of affected joints, presence of RF and HLA-B27, and clinical findings.[5] These 7 subtypes are systemic arthritis, oligoarthritis, polyarthritis (RF positive), polyarthritis (RF negative), enthesis-related arthritis (ERA), psoriatic arthritis, and undifferentiated arthritis (**Box 1**).

The authors have nothing to disclose.
[a] Department of Radiology, Miami Children's Hospital, 2100 Southwest 62nd Avenue, Miami, FL 33155, USA
[b] Department of Radiology, Children's Hospital Boston and Harvard Medical School, 300 Longwood Avenue, Boston, MA 02115, USA
* Corresponding author.
E-mail address: Ricardo.Restrepo@mch.com

Orthop Clin N Am 43 (2012) 213–225
doi:10.1016/j.ocl.2012.01.006
0030-5898/12/$ – see front matter © 2012 Published by Elsevier Inc.

> **Box 1**
> **Juvenile idiopathic arthritis classification**
>
> Systemic arthritis
>
> Oligoarthritis
>
> Polyarthritis (RF positive)
>
> Polyarthritis (RF negative)
>
> Enthesis-related arthritis
>
> Psoriatic arthritis
>
> Undifferentiated arthritis

Systemic Juvenile Idopathic Arthtitis

Systemic JIA (sJIA) constitutes a small proportion (10%) of JIA but contributes to approximately two-thirds of the total mortality rate of JIA.[7] sJIA has a prevalence of 3.5 per 100,000 and the range of incidence is between 0.4 and 0.9 per 100,00. sJIA is characterized by a preceding fever of at least 2 weeks' duration and an association with one of the following: rash, lymphadenopathy, hepatosplenomegaly, or serositis. It demonstrates no gender predilection.[6] The number of joints affected in patients with sJIA varies, and the arthritis may develop after the systemic symptoms have subsided. Although by definition, sJIA can present at any age before age 16 years, in a recent study, Behrens and colleagues[8] reported that from a total of 136 patients, 74 presented with sJIA between 0 and 5 years of age with 2 years old the most common age at presentation (n = 7). Patients affected with sJIA characteristically display early joint destructive changes and ankylosis.[2,5,6,9]

Oligoarthritis

Oligoarthritis is a term used to describe arthritis affecting 1 to 4 joints during the first 6 months of disease. Three exclusion criteria for a diagnosis of oligoarthritis are family history of psoriasis/spondyloarthropathy, positive RF, and presence of HLA-B27. Oligoarthritis is divided into 2 subcategories, persistent and extended types. The persistent type of oligoarthritis affects no more than 4 joints over the course of the illness and is more common in girls younger than 6 years of age. Monoarthritis is seen in 50% of the affected patients with the knees, ankles, and elbows as the most frequently affected joints in these children.[6] The extended type of oligoarthritis affects more than 4 joints after the first 6-month period. This subtype has a poorer prognosis than the persistent type, because more than 50% of affected patients develop the active disease in their adulthood.[6] A characteristic clinical feature of the extended type of oligoarthritis of JIA is the increased risk of iritis, especially in girls with positive antinuclear antibodies (ANAs).[2,5,6] In North America and Europe, oligoarticular disease accounts for 30% to 60% of JIA cases.[10]

Polyarthritis

Polyarthritis is a term designated for arthritis that affects 5 or more joints during the first 6 months of disease. The 2 subtypes of polyarthritis are RF positive and RF negative, the former accounting for 5% to 10% and the latter 10% to 30% of all JIA.[10] In order to establish a definite diagnosis of the RF-positive subtype of polyarthritis, it must be confirmed on 2 separate occasions that are at least 3 months apart. The RF-positive subtype of polyarthritis often begins in late childhood or adolescence and is similar to adult rheumatoid arthritis with respect to clinical presentation and pathogenesis; however, the effects on the growing skeleton (accelerated or delayed growth) make up the major difference.[2,5,6]

Enthesis-Related Arthritis

ERA is a subtype of arthritis that may be present alongside oligoarthritis or polyarthritis, affecting large or small joints as well as entheses. In addition, at least 2 of the following conditions must be present: sacroiliac pain, inflammatory lumbosacral pain, acute anterior uveitis, positivity for the HLA-B27 antigen, family history of uveitis, ankylosing spondylitis, Reiter syndrome or inflammatory bowel disease, and onset of oligoarthritis in boys over 6 years of age. Because ERA often begins as an undifferentiated disease in pediatric patients with an initial clinical presentation that differs significantly from that in adults, a definite diagnosis is frequently delayed. In contrast to adult patients with ERA, back pain is typically lacking in children with ERA and more cases of enthesopathy with knee and hip involvement are found in children (**Fig. 1**). Using the ILAR classification, most childhood spondyloarthropathies are classified as ERA and the presence of, or a family history, of psoriasis is an exclusion criterion, which differs from criteria of adult patients with ERA.[5,6,11,12]

Psoriatic Arthritis

Psoriatic arthritis is a subtype of JIA that is currently diagnosed when arthritis occurs in the presence of psoriasis or the presence of 2 of the following in conjunction with arthritis: a family history of psoriasis in a first-degree relative, dactylitis, and nail changes. The presence of RF is an exclusion criterion for a diagnosis of psoriatic arthritis. Accounting for approximately 5% of JIA,

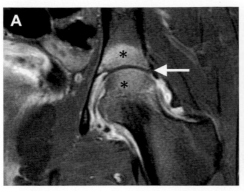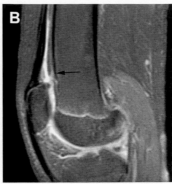

Fig. 1. A 15-year-old boy with ankylosing spondylitis. (A) Coronal T2-weighted fat-suppressed image with contrast shows a left hip joint effusion with synovitis, bone marrow edema (*asterisks*), and joint space narrowing due to diffuse cartilage loss (*arrow*). (B) Sagittal T1-weighted fat-suppressed image with contrast shows a tiny knee effusion with synovial enhancement, indicating synovitis (*arrow*).

psoriatic arthritis tends to affect girls more frequently than boys and often begins earlier in childhood.[5,6,13] It is still debated whether this subtype should be regarded as an entirely separate entity due to a heterogeneously distinct profile in children with early-onset and late-onset types. The early-onset type of psoriatic arthritis peaks at age 2 to 3 years, is more common among girls, and tends to be ANA positive with clinical features similar to oligoarticular/polyarticular JIA. The late-onset type of psoriatic arthritis, alternatively, peaks at approximately 10 to 12 years and is accompanied by features typical of spondyloarthritis, such as male predominance, HLA-B27 positivity, enthesis, and axial skeletal involvement. Both types of psoriatic arthritis are accompanied by a high frequency of dactylitis and arthritis that may precede skin manifestations.[13]

Undifferentiated Arthritis

A diagnosis of undifferentiated arthritis should be made only after careful evaluation and exclusion of other types of arthritis.[5,6]

PATHOGENESIS

Immune-mediated diseases manifest differently, depending on the underlying abnormalities of the adaptive and innate immune responses. Autoimmunity is the result of immune reactions that are triggered by environmental factors in genetically susceptible individuals. Autoimmune diseases involve the adaptive immune system and are based on antigen-dependent T-lymphocyte and B-cell autoantibody production and have strong associations with the major histocompatibility complex. Alternatively, autoinflammatory diseases causing innate immunity disorders are due to underlying mutations associated with innate immune cells,

such as monocytes and neutrophils, rather than to lymphocytes causing immune dysregulation.[9,14,15] More recently, an immunologic disease continuum has been proposed, which classifies diseases according to adaptive or innate immune responses, with the majority of diseases involving variable interactions between these 2 systems. Tissue perturbations at target sites of inflammation, rather than the immune system per se, are the key to disease expression.[15]

Oligoarticular/Polyarticular Arthritis

Currently, sufficient evidence supports a distinct pathogenesis of oligoarticular/polyarticular JIA and sJIA. Various known genetic and environmental factors are associated with the development of oligoarticular/polyarticular JIA. With respect to genetic associations, several studies have indicated specific genetic susceptibility with respect to the HLA and non-HLA types.[16] Likewise, environmental factors, such as infectious agents, stress, maternal smoking, and weather changes, as well as vaccination have been associated with the onset or exacerbation of oligoarticular/polyarticular JIA.[2,16] Oligoarticular/polyarticular JIA is believed to be an antigen-driven, lymphocyte-mediated autoimmune disease. An abnormality in the adaptive immune system, in which an imbalance exists between proinflammatory T cells (Th1 and Th17) and immunosuppressive regulatory T cells (CD4+, which play an important role in immune tolerance to self-antigen), leads to the failure of T-cell tolerance to self-antigens and eventually results in synovitis.[2,16,17]

Systemic Idiopathic Arthritis

Systemic idiopathic arthritis is an autoinflammatory disease involving the innate immune system. Unlike with oligoarticular/polyarticular disease, there is no clear association between sJIA and infection, vaccination, or HLA genes. In the early course of the disease process, unknown factors cause loss of control of the alternative secretory pathway (which differs from the classical intracellular transport mechanism), leading to the activation of phagocytes and resulting in the release of proinflammatory cytokines, macrophage colony-stimulating factor, tumor necrosis factor (TNF), and proinflammatory proteins. Such complex underlying interactions are believed to contribute to the multisystemic inflammation seen in sJIA.[9,16]

Enthesis-Related Arthritis

It is well known that genetics plays a major role in developing ERA. The classic example is patients with ankylosing spondylitis, 80% to 90% of whom are HLA-B27 positive. Not all of those patients are HLA-B27 positive, however, and not every person who has the antigen develops the disease, suggesting other associated factors. Traditionally, ERA has been thought of as an autoimmune disease, in which spondyloarthritis is triggered by gastrointestinal or urologic infections in the presence of HLA-B27– restricted CD8–T-cell clones that are reactive against bacterial antigens and self-proteins from cartilage in the inflamed joint.[18] More recently, an autoinflammatory component of the disease has been suggested, with HLA-B27 playing a role in triggering the innate immune system rather than through antigen presentation. According to this hypothesis, the HLA-B27 molecule may be prone to misfolding within the endoplasmic reticulum of the cell, resulting in the stimulation of the innate immune system, with a greater impact on tissues exposed to either bacterial or mechanical stress, such as the gut and synovium.[14,18] The concept of a synovial-entheseal complex proposed by Benjamin and McGonagle[19] suggests a relationship between synovial-entheseal complex and spondyloarthropathies. This concept is based on entheses as sites of repeated biomechanical stress that undergo chronic microtrauma, causing the release of fibronectin and other molecules from the injured tissue. These molecules may activate synovial macrophages, resulting in the activation of stress-related genes. Other genetic factors have been identified, such as polymorphism in or near the TNF and interleukin-1 and interleukin-23 loci. These cytokines play an important role in the propagation and perpetuation of inflammation in spondyloarthropathies, providing additional evidence for the innate immune system's contribution to ERA.[14,18]

Psoriatic Arthritis

As discussed previously regarding classification of arthritis, there are 2 subtypes of the disease, based not only on different ages of onset but also on the underlying pathogenesis. The disease with the older onset shares features with spondyloarthropathies and, as such, has a similar pathogenesis. Innate immunologic mechanisms likely play a role in the older-onset psoriatic JIA, which typically manifests as inflammation of either the entheses, the intestinal tract, or both and is ultimately responsible for the synovitis.[13,14,18,19] The early-onset subtype of psoriatic arthritis is more likely associated with HLA alleles with early presentation, ANA positivity, and chronic uveitis rather than with HLA-B27. The association suggests that adaptive immunity is more involved than it is in older-onset patients. One feature that remains unexplained is the presence of dactylitis, which is only seen in both subtypes of psoriatic JIA, thus suggesting that both adaptive immunologic and innate autoinflammatory mechanisms are involved in this type of arthritis.[13]

IMAGING EVALUATION AND SPECTRUM OF IMAGING FINDINGS

When imaging pediatric patients with JIA, it is important to understand the underlying disease

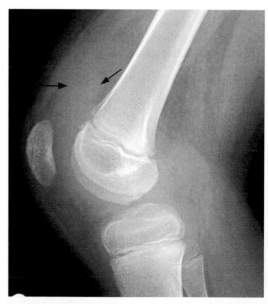

Fig. 2. A 9-year-old girl with 2 episodes of atraumatic prolonged painful knee swelling in the preceding 6 months. Lateral radiograph of the knee shows a suprapatellar effusion (*arrows*). The frontal radiograph was negative (not shown).

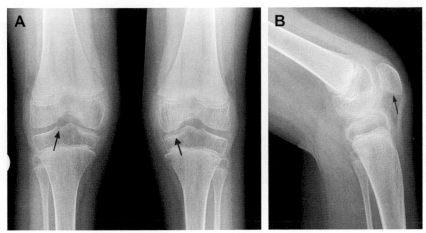

Fig. 3. A 13-year-old girl with RF-positive JIA. (*A*) Frontal radiograph of both knees shows severe osteopenia and erosive changes of the tibial articular surface (*arrows*). (*B*) Lateral radiograph shows ballooning of the femoral epiphysis and squaring of the patella (*arrow*).

process. The hallmark of JIA is synovial inflammation that manifests clinically as painful joint swelling associated with a limited range of motion. Acute synovitis, which progresses to chronic synovitis, can lead to synovial hypertrophy, resulting in soft tissue swelling and joint fluid accumulation. Subsequently, highly cellular pannus forms and spreads from the periphery to the center of the joint, resulting in eventual damage of the cartilage, cortical bone, and, finally, the underlying bone marrow. These cartilage and bone lesions represent the late and irreversible joint changes in patients affected with JIA.[20,21]

Currently, there are no universally accepted imaging protocols for JIA. The selection of imaging modality used varies from patient to patient and according to the timing of the visit, such as in patients with an acutely swollen knee or with a known diagnosis of JIA. In patients with an acutely swollen knee joint, imaging takes on the complementary role of excluding other processes, such as a septic joint, and narrowing the differential diagnosis. Diagnosis of JIA is entirely clinically based, as defined by ILAR.[5] With confirmed JIA, imaging studies are usually obtained for patients with worsening symptoms to monitor disease progression or treatment response and to evaluate complications.

Conventional Radiography

Plain radiographs are frequently the initial imaging modality obtained in evaluation of JIA. Although radiographs are not diagnostic, they often provide useful clues toward diagnosis of disease and help exclude other joint diseases. In cases of confirmed JIA, plain radiographs often demonstrate soft tissue swelling, joint effusions (**Fig. 2**), periarticular osteopenia, periosteal reaction, epiphyseal remodeling, knee joint space narrowing, and cartilage/bone erosions (**Fig. 3**). Signs of advanced skeletal maturity, such as early physeal fusion and leg length discrepancy, are complications that can be seen on radiographs.[21] Radiographs

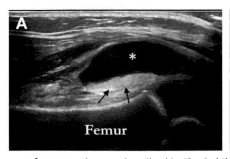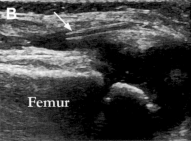

Fig. 4. US images of same patient as described in **Fig. 2**. (*A*) Sagittal grayscale US image of the knee shows a large effusion (*asterisk*) and nodular thickening of the synovium, indicating synovitis (*arrows*). (*B*) Sagittal US image shows near-complete resolution of the effusion after arthrocentesis. The tip of the needle (*arrow*) is visualized in the joint space.

A   **B**

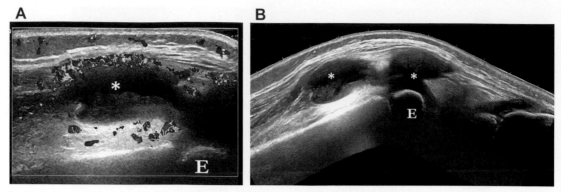

Fig. 5. A 6-year-old girl with RF-positive JIA. (*A*) Color Doppler image shows a joint effusion (*asterisk*) with marked hyperemia of the synovium, indicating active inflammation. (*B*) Panoramic view of the knee (extended field of view) shows the extent of the effusion (*asterisks*). E, epiphysis.

have been used for disease staging and evaluating disease progression.[21–25] Early on in the disease, however, radiographs can appear normal due to the predominantly cartilaginous pediatric knee and the inability to demonstrate synovitis or to differentiate it from a joint effusion. Scoring systems based on radiographs for evaluating the degree of joint destruction have significant inter-reader and intrareader variability.[23,26] Although assessing structural damage to joints over time is essential in evaluating treatment response and disease progression, early radiographic changes are not specific. Furthermore, radiographic scoring systems are based on adult rheumatoid arthritis and are inadequate for measuring changes in the growing joint.[25] Routine follow-up radiographs of a specific joint are not indicated, because they are poor predictors of disease activity due to the slow development of findings. Consequently, a careful assessment of clinical symptoms and physical examination are of paramount importance.[21,24,27]

Ultrasound and Color Doppler

Well-known advantages of ultrasound (US), particularly for pediatric patients, include wide availability, lack of radiation, portability, no sedation required and multiple joints can be evaluated simultaneously. Improved resolution, particularly with the high-frequency transducers that are currently available in new US machines, allows visualization of detailed intra-articular structures and the soft tissues. On US, the presence and degree of synovial thickening, the size of the effusion (**Fig. 4**A), the presence of popliteal cysts, and adenopathy can be evaluated.[21,28,29] Doppler interrogation can enable the detection of synovial and soft tissue hyperemia (**Fig. 5**). US can been used to guide the needle aspiration

of a knee effusion (see **Fig. 4**B) as well as to evaluate disease activity and/or response to therapy. Early US findings that are suggestive of disease progression are an increase in the amount of fluid followed by increased and more extensive synovial thickening. On color Doppler, the US finding of decreasing vascularity is suggestive of improving synovitis (**Fig. 6**).[21,28–30] Limitations of US in evaluating the knee include an inability to assess the entire joint and to evaluate cartilage thickness and erosions in certain parts of the joint as skeletal maturation progresses.

MRI

MRI provides a comprehensive evaluation of articular cartilage, bone marrow, cortical bone, and soft tissues changes with the progression of the disease. MRI not only can evaluate the entire articular

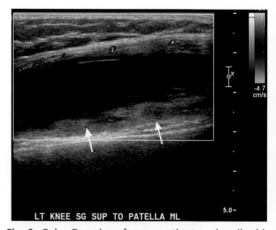

LT KNEE SG SUP TO PATELLA ML

Fig. 6. Color Doppler of same patient as described in Fig. 5 after 6 months of treatment with methotrexate shows a decrease in the joint effusion and improvement of the synovial thickening (*arrows*) and hyperemia.

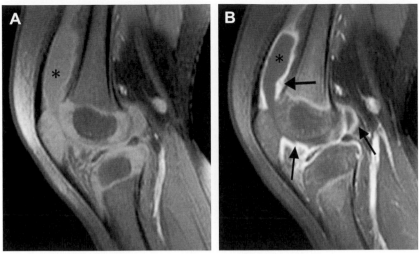

Fig. 7. A 4-year-old girl with oligoarticular JIA presented initially with swollen and painful knee. Sagittal T1-weighted image with fat saturation before (*A*) and after (*B*) IV contrast shows a very large joint effusion (*asterisks*) and synovial enhancement (*arrows*), indicating synovitis only after IV contrast administration. A popliteal lymph node is present.

cartilage but also can help differentiate it from the epiphyseal growth cartilage. Similar to US, MRI can confidently differentiate a proliferative synovial thickening/pannus from a joint effusion. MRI has the capability to detect disease at an earlier stage and to evaluate disease progression, thereby potentially having an impact on management and prognosis.[29,30] In order to identify underlying synovial inflammation and to differentiate it from a joint effusion, intravenous gadolinium is usually necessary (**Fig. 7**). MRI must be acquired immediately after contrast injection because gadolinium diffuses into the joint fluid; thus, only one joint can be imaged at a time. Due to its capacity to evaluate cortical bone and marrow, MRI is particularly useful in identifying bone erosions in early stages. Early MRI findings in JIA include hypertrophic enhancing synovium, soft tissue edema, irregularity of the infrapatellar fat pad, and popliteal lymphadenopathy (**Fig. 8**).[20,21,31] Drawbacks to MRI are the expensive cost, the time required to conduct the study, and the possible need for sedating younger children.[28,29] In a recent study, MRI was found useful in differentiating subtypes of recent-onset childhood arthritis,

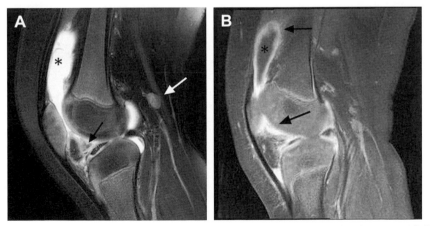

Fig. 8. A 3-year-old boy recently diagnosed with psoriatic JIA. (*A*) Sagittal T2-weighted image with fat saturation shows a large joint effusion (*asterisk*), edema, and stranding of Hoffa fat pad (*black arrow*) as well as a popliteal adenopathy (*white arrow*). (*B*) Sagittal T1-weighted fat-saturated image with gadolinium differentiates the joint effusion (*asterisk*) from the synovitis, seen as thickening and enhancement of the synovium (*arrows*).

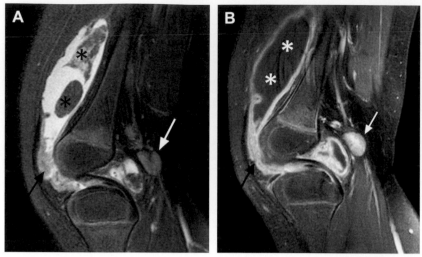

Fig. 9. A 7-year-old girl with pauciarticular JIA presented with a warm, painful, and swollen knee. (*A*) Sagittal T2-weighted image with fat saturation shows joint effusion containing hypointensities (*asterisks*) and irregular synovial thickening (*black arrow*). Popliteal adenopathy is present (*white arrow*). (*B*) Corresponding T1-weighted image after IV gadolinium shows synovial enhancement (*black arrow*) but no contrast enhancement of the intra-articular hypointensities (*asterisks*). Popliteal adenopathy is seen (*white arrow*).

such as infectious arthritis, postinfectious arthritis, and JIA, which can have a therapeutic effect on patients with an acutely swollen knee. In this study, irregular synovial thickening as well as nonenhancing low T2 signal synovial tissue (**Fig. 9**) were found as early and differentiating features supporting JIA rather than other types of arthritis.[32] Gradient sequences are routinely used to detect hemosiderin

in cases of pigmented villonodular synovitis, which presents with joint effusion and synovitis. Because of a blooming artifact, however, very dark areas are seen if hemosiderin is present (**Fig. 10**).[33] Although several studies have suggested MRI for evaluating JIA, even in the early stages, in a study by Miller and colleagues,[34] only fair evidence was found to support MRI as an accurate diagnostic

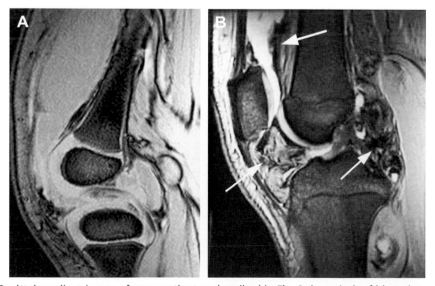

Fig. 10. (*A*) Sagittal gradient image of same patient as described in **Fig. 9** shows lack of blooming artifact in the joint effusion. (*B*) Sagittal gradient image in an adolescent boy with pigmented villonodular synovitis shows blooming artifact as dark areas in Hoffa fat, suprapatellar bursa, and posterior intercondylar regions, indicating the presence of hemosiderin (*arrows*).

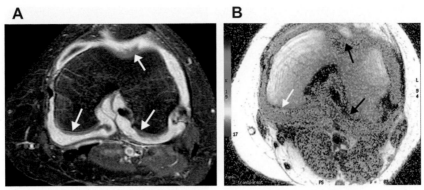

Fig. 11. T2 mapping in a patient with polyarticular JIA. (*A*) Axial T1-weighted image with gadolinium shows uniform enhancement of thick pannus (*bright areas*) surrounding the femoral condyles (*arrows*). The subtle irregularity of the articular cartilage is indicative of early cartilage lesions. (*B*) T2 mapping image at the same level shows more green and blue in the articular cartilage, indicating abnormal T2 relaxation values of both femoral condyles and trochlear groove cartilage (*arrows*).

method to evaluate synovium or cartilage and clinical response to treatment in peripheral joints, including the knee. More recently, MRI has been used to study cartilage physiology and biochemistry. One of the earliest physiologic changes in cartilage degeneration is increased permeability, which leads to increased water content, resulting in increased stress and eventual cartilage degeneration. T2 relaxation time mapping has been shown effective in detecting early physiologic and microstructural changes in the cartilage before morphologic changes are detected on conventional MRI. The T2 relaxation value is a constant for a given tissue (ie, articular cartilage) that changes with tissue

damage.[35,36] Specifically, in patients with JIA, higher T2 relaxation times have been found when compared with healthy subjects, demonstrating the usefulness of cartilage T2 mapping for the early detection of microstructural changes in JIA (**Fig. 11**).[37]

Spectrum of Imaging Findings of Juvenile Idiopathic Arthritis

Synovitis

On US, synovitis is seen as a thickening and nodularity of the synovium with increased vascularity in cases of active inflammation. On MRI, normal synovium is smooth, is up to 2 mm thick, and

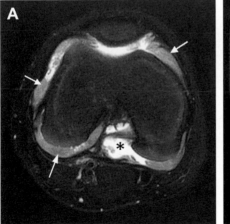
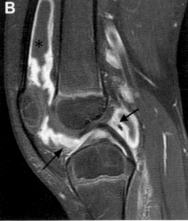

Fig. 12. A 16-year-old girl receiving treatment of RF-positive JIA complains of progressive flexure contracture of the knee. (*A*) Axial T2-weighted image shows severe pannus formation surrounding the femoral condyles (*arrows*) and a joint effusion (*asterisk*). (*B*) Sagittal T1-weighted image with fat saturation after IV gadolinium shows vivid enhancement of the thick pannus in the intercondylar notch surrounding the anterior cruciate ligament (*arrows*), which limits the range of motion. Joint effusion (*asterisk*) is also seen.

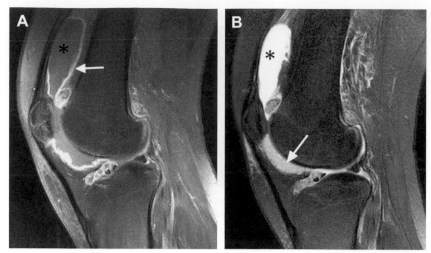

Fig. 13. A 17-year-old girl with RF-positive JIA presents with decreasing range of motion. (*A*) Sagittal T1-weighted image with contrast shows a large joint effusion (*asterisk*) and synovitis (*arrow*). (*B*) Sagittal T2-weighted image with fat saturation shows multiple tiny foci of signal intensity similar to cartilage (*arrow*). These tiny foci were not discernible on the T1 sequence and seem consistent with cartilaginous loose bodies. A hyperintense large supra-patellar joint effusion (*asterisk*).

displays minimal contrast enhancement. In contrast, inflamed synovium is irregular and thickened with increased signal intensity, allowing a clear distinction between pannus, effusion, and articular cartilage (**Fig. 12**). In acute and/or active synovitis, the contrast enhancement is diffuse and homogeneous, whereas the enhancement of fibrotic inactive synovium tends to be mild, patchy, and heterogeneous.[21,28,29] Fluid-sensitive MRI

sequences allow for the detection of rice bodies as dark structures, surrounded by the brighter fluid that occasionally occur in JIA (**Fig. 13**).[21,28–30,38]

Articular cartilage, bone marrow, and joint space

MRI is an excellent imaging modality for evaluating intra-articular cartilage signal intensity changes, including focal lesions, in a joint. MRI can detect

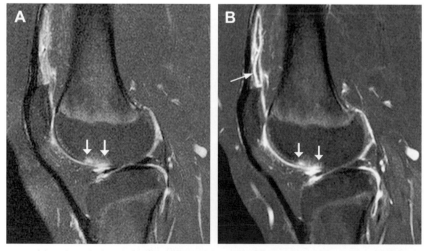

Fig. 14. A 15-year-old girl with longstanding RF-positive JIA. (*A*) Sagittal STIR image shows 2 osteochondral erosions in the lateral femoral condyle with extension into the subchondral bone (*arrows*). (*B*) Sagittal T1-weighted fat-suppressed image with contrast shows enhancement of the erosions (*short white arrows*) and evidence of synovitis (*long white arrow*). A lymph node is seen in the popliteal fossa. Radiographs (not shown) did not reveal an abnormality.

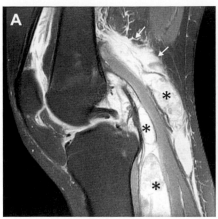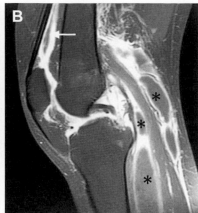

Fig. 15. A 16-year-old boy with oligoarticular JIA. (*A*) Sagittal T2-weighted image shows a joint effusion, soft tissue edema (*arrows*), and a multiloculated popliteal cyst with hypointense material (*asterisks*). (*B*) Sagittal T1-weighted fat-suppressed image with contrast shows a small joint effusion (*arrow*) and the multiloculated popliteal cyst (*asterisks*) with enhancing synovium, indicating synovitis.

early subtle changes in the articular cartilage, such as thinning and focal chondral defects, particularly on postcontrast T1-weighted image fat-saturated sequences. Erosions are not a constant finding in JIA, tend to occur late in the disease, and are more frequently seen with RF-positive polyarthritis. Erosions indicate destruction of underlying cartilage and bone and more often, although not exclusively, occur at the insertion sites of ligaments and tendons and at the sites of synovial reflection. In cases of juvenile psoriatic arthritis, multifocal enhancing bone marrow edema at articular and nonarticular sites has been described.[39] Radiographs tend to underestimate the underlying osseous erosive changes, because they are relatively insensitive to trabecular bone loss, which is most significantly affected by erosion (**Fig. 14**). Generalized joint space narrowing is an indirect sign that reflects a more uniform cartilage loss.[21] A recent study found good agreement between US and MRI with respect to quantifying the thickness of the knee cartilage, with a better reproducibility with the MRI. This study only included prepubertal children, who have more cartilaginous knees with better US windows. The need for age-related and gender-related standard reference values for articular cartilage thickness on US in healthy children came to light, as has previously been determined for the metacarpophalangeal and interphalangeal joints.[40,41] On US, bony erosions are defined as cortical defects that are larger than 2 mm and that have an irregular floor seen in 2 planes.[42] Medial meniscal hypoplasia is a well-known finding in patients with JIA, presumably due to the extension of the hypertrophic synovium over the meniscal surface.[21]

Soft tissues

Several soft tissue abnormalities around the knee have been described in patients with JIA. These findings are best evaluated on US or MRI, because with their limited capability, radiographs play virtually no role in their evaluation. Soft tissue abnormalities are nonspecific for the disease and include stranding and edema of the infrapatellar fat pad, popliteal cysts (**Fig. 15**), adenopathy, enthesitis, tenosynovitis, and hypoplasia of the cruciate ligaments. Among these findings, the only one that seems useful as a secondary sign of inflammation in early JIA is the inflammation of the infrapatellar fat pad, which is best seen on MRI (see **Fig. 8**).[31] Popliteal lymphadenopathy, although not pathognomonic, is frequently seen in JIA (see **Fig. 8**).[20,21]

SUMMARY

JIA refers to a group of chronic arthritic conditions arising before 16 years of age. Although the term is not perfect, it has been useful clinically and for research purposes. To date, there is still significant morbidity associated with JIA during childhood and adolescence, and challenges for the future include early identification of those with a poorer prognosis. There are currently no established guidelines in imaging JIA; however, imaging can play a complementary role in selected cases. Evidence indicates that radiographs play only a small role once a diagnosis has been made, leaving US and MRI as imaging modalities of choice for answering specific questions pertaining to disease classification, staging, and outcome of treatment options. Improvements in MRI, including the use of higher field strength systems and improved cartilage sequences, seem promising and may be of significant value in the near future. More aggressive and more specific therapies for JIA demand a prompt diagnosis at an early stage of the disease and an accurate evaluation of response to treatment to have an impact on the outcome of the disease. Although the ILAR classification is imperfect, it is an important step in the unification of terminology, understanding of the disease, and treatment. Diagnosis of JIA is clinically based; however, clinical and laboratory findings have demonstrated poor sensitivity in assessing disease activity. An imaging scoring system focusing on MRI or US that addresses early rather than late and irreversible radiographic changes should be developed in an effort to further standardize and evaluate disease progression as well as treatment response.

REFERENCES

1. Murray K, Thompson SD, Glass DN. Pathogenesis of juvenile chronic arthritis: genetic and environmental factors. Arch Dis Child 1997;77:530–4.
2. Prakken B, Albani S, Martini A. Juvenile idiopathic arthritis. Lancet 2011;377:2138–49.
3. Manners PJ, Bower C. Worldwide prevalence of juvenile arthritis why does it vary so much? J Rheumatol 2002;29:1520–30.
4. Saurenmann K, Rose JB, Tyrell P, et al. Epidemiology of juvenile idiopathic arthritis in a multiethnic cohort: ethnicity as a risk factor. Arthritis Rheum 2007;56:1974–84.
5. Petty RE, Southwood TR, Manners P, et al. International League of Associations for Rheumatology classification of juvenile idiopathic arthritis: second revision, Edmonton. J Rheumatol 2004;31:390–2.
6. Jordan A, McDonagh JE. Juvenile idiopathic arthritis: the pediatric perspective. Pediatr Radiol 2006;36:734–42.
7. Gurion R, Lehman TJ, Moorthy LN. Systemic arthritis in children: a review of clinical presentation and treatment. Int J Inflam 2012;2012:271569. [Epub 2011 Dec 25].
8. Behrens EM, Beukelman T, Gallo L, et al. Evaluation of the presentation of systemic onset juvenile rheumatoid arthritis: data from the Pennsylvania Systemic Onset Juvenile Arthritis Registry (PASO-JAR). J Rheumatol 2008;35:343–8.
9. Mellins E, Macaubas C, Grom A. Pathogenesis of systemic juvenile idiopathic arthritis: some answers, more questions. Nat Rev Rheumatol 2011;7:416–26.
10. Ravelli A, Martini A. Juvenile idiopahtic arthritis. Lancet 2007;369:767–78.
11. Colbert RA. Classification of juvenile spondyloarthritis: enthesis related arthritis and beyond. Nat Rev Rheumatol 2010;6:477–85.
12. Hofer M. Spondyloarthropathies in children—are they different from those in adults? Best Pract Res Clin Rheumatol 2006;20:315–28.
13. Stoll ML, Punaro M. Psoriatic juvenile idiopathic arthritis: a tale of two subgroups. Curr Opin Rheumatol 2011;23:1–7.
14. Stoll ML. Interactions of the innate and adaptive arms of the immune system in the pathogenesis of spondyloarthritis. Clin Exp Rheumatol 2011;29:322–30.
15. Mcgonagle D, Aziz A, Dickie LJ, et al. An integrated classification of pediatric inflammatory diseases based on the concepts of autoinflammation and the immunological disease continuum. Pediatr Res 2009;65:38R–45R.
16. Lin UT, Wang CT, Gershwin ME, et al. The pathogenesis of oligoarticular/polyarticular vs systemic juvenile idiopathic arthritis. Autoimmun Rev 2011;10:482–9.
17. Macaubas C, Nguyen K, Milojevic D, et al. Oligoarticular and polyarticular JIA: epidemiology and pathogenesis. Nat Rev Rheumatol 2009;5:616–26.
18. Dougados M, Baeten D. Spondyloarthritis. Lancet 2011;377:2127–37.
19. Benjamin M, McGonagle D. The enthesis organ concept and its relevance to the spondyloarthropathies. Adv Exp Med Biol 2009;649:57–70.
20. Johnson K, Wittkop B, Haigh F, et al. The early magnetic resonance imaging features of juvenile idiopathic arthritis. Clin Radiol 2002;57:466–71.
21. Johnson K. Imaging of juvenile idiopathic arthritis. Pediatr Radiol 2006;36:743–58.
22. Pettersson H, Rydolm U. Radiologic classification of knee joint destruction in juvenile chronic arthritis. Pediatr Radiol 1984;14:419–21.
23. Doria AS, de Castro CC, Kiss MH, et al. Inter and intrareader variability in the interpretation of two radiographic classification systems for juvenile rheumatoid arthritis. Pediatr Radiol 2003;33:673–81.
24. Oen K, Reed M, Mallerson PN, et al. Radiologic outcome and its relationship to functional disability in juvenile rheumatoid arthritis. J Rheumatol 2003;30:832–40.
25. Doria AS, Babyn PS, Feldman B. A critical appraisal of radiographic scoring systems for assessment of juvenile idiopathic arthritis. Pediatr Radiol 2006;36:759–72.
26. Johnson K. Commentary on "inter and intrareader variability in the interpretation of two radiographic classification systems for juvenile rheumatoid arthritis." Pediatr Radiol 2003;33:671–2.
27. Johnson K, Gardner-Medwin J. Childhood arthritis: classification and radiology. Clin Radiol 2002;57:47–58.
28. Sureda D, Quiroga S, Arnal C, et al. Juvenile rheumatoid arthritis of the knee. Evaluation with US. Radiology 1994;190:403–6.

29. Lamer S, Sebag GH. MRI and ultrasound in children with juvenile chronic arthritis. Eur J Radiol 2000;33: 85–93.

30. Cellerini M, Salti S, Trapani S, et al. Correlation between clinical and ultrasound assessment of the knee in children with mono-articular or pauci-articular juvenile rheumatoid arthritis. Pediatr Radiol 1999;29:117–23.

31. Gylys-Morin V, Graham TB, Blebea JS, et al. Knee in early juvenile rheumatoid arthritis: imaging findings. Radiology 2001;220:696–706.

32. Kirkhus E, Flato B, Riise O, et al. Differences in MRI findings between subgroups of recent-onset childhood arthritis. Pediatr Radiol 2011;41:432–40.

33. Hughes TH, Sartoris DJ, Schweitzer ME. Pigmented villonodular synovitis: MRI characteristics. Skeletal Radiol 1995;24:7–12.

34. Miller E, Uleryk E, Doria A. Evidence-based outcomes of studies addressing diagnostic accuracy of MRI of juvenile idiopathic arthritis. AJR Am J Roentgenol 2009;192:1209–18.

35. Kim HK, Laor T, Graham TB. T2 relaxation time changes in distal femoral articular cartilage in children with juvenile idiopathic arthritis: a 3-year longitudinal study. AJR Am J Roentgenol 2010;195: 1021–5.

36. Choi JA, Gold GE. MR imaging of articular cartilage physiology. Magn Reson Imaging Clin N Am 2011; 19:249–82.

37. Knight AC, Dardzinski BJ, Laor T, et al. Magnetic resonance imaging evaluation of the effects of juvenile rheumatoid arthritis on distal femoral weight-bearing cartilage. Arthritis Rheum 2004;50:901–5.

38. Chung C, Coley BD, Martin LC. Rice bodies in juvenile rheumatoid arthritis. AJR Am J Roentgenol 1998;170:698–700.

39. Lee EY, Sundel RP, Kim S, et al. MRI findings of juvenile psoriatic arthritis. Skeletal Radiol 2008;37:987–96.

40. Spannow AH, Stenboeg E, Pfeiffer-Jensen M, et al. Ultrasound and MRI measurements of joint cartilage in healthy children: a validation study. Ultraschall Med 2011;32:s110–6.

41. Spannow AH, Pfeiffer-Jensen M, Andresen NT, et al. Ultrasonographic measurements of joint cartilage thickness in healthy children: age- and sex-related standard reference values. J Rheumatol 2010;37: 2595–601.

42. Wakkefield RJ, Gibbon WW, Conaghan PG, et al. The value of sonography in the detection of bone erosions in patients with rheumatoid arthritis: a comparison with conventional radiography. Arthritis Rheum 2000;43:2762–70.

Acute Traumatic and Sports-Related Osteochondral Injury of the Pediatric Knee

Dennis E. Kramer, MD*, J. Lee Pace, MD

KEYWORDS

- Pediatric • Knee • Osteochondral fragments • Hemarthrosis
- Patellar dislocation

Acute traumatic and sports-related osteochondral (OC) injuries occur in a variety of settings in the pediatric knee. The pediatric population is more susceptible to OC fractures because the calcified cartilage layer is incompletely formed, which results in a weakened interface between the articular cartilage and subchondral bone.[1,2] OC fractures occur in the patella or trochlea of children after a noncontact flexion-rotation injury to the knee, which results in an acute patellar dislocation. Such injuries can also occur in the femoral condyles after a patellar dislocation or either a contact or noncontact injury to the knee, causing a shearing force on the condyles. Acute OC fractures should be addressed surgically in cases where the OC fragment is large and the donor site is in a weight-bearing area.

OC injuries can lead to progressive chondral damage and early-onset arthritis. There is a small-window of time in which surgical repair of the loose OC fragment is optimal. Over time, the loose OC fragment swells and chondral degeneration occurs. In addition, the loose fragment can damage other chondral surfaces in the knee. Early surgical repair of a large intact OC fragment has the potential to restore anatomy and preserve the native chondral surface. When the fragment is deemed unsalvageable, the loose body is removed and the donor site is treated with cartilage resurfacing techniques, such as microfracture, OC plugs, and autologous chondrocyte implantation (ACI).[3,4] These techniques generate repair tissue with inferior histologic and long-term wear characteristics compared with the native chondral surface.

BACKGROUND AND MECHANISM OF OC FRACTURE DURING PATELLAR DISLOCATION

Acute lateral patellar dislocations are the most common cause of OC fractures in the pediatric knee. A noncontact flexion-rotation injury to the knee causes the patella to dislocate laterally and shear across the lateral femoral condyle (LFC). Impaction of the medial border of the patella to the LFC/trochlea during patellar relocation results in the fracture.[2] OC fractures occur in 25% to 75% of acute patellar dislocations in the pediatric and adolescent population.[5–8] These injuries most often involve the medial facet of the patella[9] and are missed on standard radiographs in up to 36% of cases.[2,6] Two studies emphasized how common OC injuries can be after acute patellar dislocations. Using radiography and arthroscopy, Stanitski and Paletta[8] assessed articular lesions in 48 pediatric patients (24 male and 24 female; mean age 14 years) with acute, initial, noncontact patellar dislocations. Of 48 patients, they identified arthroscopically 32 patients with OC fractures and 2 patients with chondral injuries as well as 28 patients with OC loose bodies. Only 32% of the

The authors have nothing to disclose.
Division of Sports Medicine, Department of Orthopaedic Surgery, Children's Hospital Boston, Harvard Medical School, 300 Longwood Avenue, Boston, MA 02115, USA
* Corresponding author.
E-mail address: Dennis.kramer@childrens.harvard.edu

arthroscopically visualized OC/chondral lesions were noted on preoperative radiographs. Nomura and colleagues[10] arthroscopically evaluated the knees of 39 pediatric patients with initial lateral patellar dislocation. Knees of 37 of their 39 patients (95%) had a chondral injury, including 28 patients with OC fractures, which were most commonly noted at the medial patellar facet.

OC fractures of the weight-bearing femoral condyles can present in isolation or in the setting of a traumatic patellar dislocation.[11–13] This fracture is rare and occurs almost exclusively in the LFC. Two studies reported a rate of 8% and 20% for OC fractures of the associated weight-bearing LFC with patellar dislocations.[10,14] Both studies were small in number, and the study by Nomura and colleagues[10] included patients up to the age of 40 years with 72% of patients aged 12 to 19 years. OC fractures of the medial femoral condyle (MFC) are rare and are only described as case reports in the literature.[11,15–19] Review of these articles shows that more of these injuries are in the non–weight-bearing portion of the MFC. Bowers and Huffman[19] reported an MFC fracture after a forced hyperextension injury in a 25-year-old woman. Occult subcortical and/or depression fractures of the femoral condyles have also been described.[20–22] These injuries can occur in isolation or in combination with a ligamentous injury.

Similar to OC injuries in the trochlea, the postulated mechanism for weight-bearing condylar fractures in association with a patellar dislocation is when the relocating patella directly impacts the femoral condyle, producing fracture. The difference is thought to be the degree of knee flexion present during injury. Knee flexion at 90° or more at the time of dislocation and/or relocation are thought to be present for this injury pattern.[23] In isolation, a valgus-shearing mechanism coupled with a twist between the femoral condyle and the tibial plateau is thought to occur.[11,13] This latter mechanism has also been proposed to explain the weight-bearing OC condyle fracture even in association with patellar dislocations, given the highly constrained nature of the patella when the knee is highly flexed.[12] These injuries are typically noncontact. This mechanism is applicable mainly to LFC fractures. MFC fractures are so rare that no clear mechanism has been described. Generalized joint hypermobility may be a risk factor for the occurrence of this injury.[13,24]

CLINICAL PRESENTATION AND DIAGNOSIS

An acute patellar dislocation with an associated OC injury can occur after both traumatic contact and noncontact twisting injuries to the knee. Patients often present with a large knee effusion, tenderness over the medial retinaculum/medial patellofemoral ligament, and lateral patellar subluxation. The effusion, if aspirated, reveals a lipohemarthrosis resulting from the OC fracture. Range of motion may or may not be significantly disturbed depending on the location of the loose OC fragment. Often, the fragment can end up in the suprapatellar pouch or in one of the gutters. Significant crepitus of the area may be appreciated on range of motion. Patients often are unable to bear weight. The examiner should assess for ligament integrity and an intact extensor mechanism.

Lateral, sunrise, and Merchant-view radiographs of the knee may be helpful in identifying loose bodies and assessing pertinent anatomic factors, such as patella alta and trochlear dysplasia (**Fig. 1**). In patients with a large hemarthrosis and a traumatic mechanism, the clinician should have a strong suspicion for OC injury. Initial radiographs can be misleading. Often they are negative or show only a small fleck of bone.[13,25]

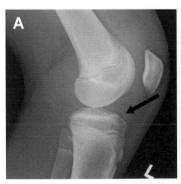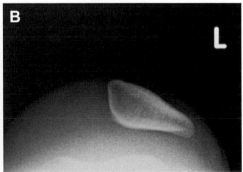

Fig. 1. Lateral (*A*) and Merchant-view (*B*) radiographs of a 14-year-old patient showing a patellar dislocation when relocated. Note an acute OC fracture (*black arrow*) visible on the lateral view.

Nonstandard oblique views may be needed to appreciate the OC fragment.[25] If radiographs do not reveal any loose bodies, further imaging may be indicated. Magnetic resonance imaging (MRI) is typically the study of choice for high-resolution scanning and evaluation of OC lesions.[14,25] Improved MR protocols using intravenous gadolinium and appropriate orthogonal tilting on a 1.5-T magnet have increased MRI sensitivity and specificity to 90% to 95% for localizing and characterizing OC injuries (**Fig. 2**).[26–30] MRI may underestimate the true size of the defect because the partially attached chondral fragments have an irregular shape that may not correspond to the plane of the image.[26] Computed tomography (CT) may also be used to better visualize the donor site and loose fragment as well as plan the operative management (**Fig. 3**). Arthroscopy remains the gold standard for the accurate identification and characterization of OC injuries.

MANAGEMENT AND SURGICAL TECHNIQUE

Nonoperative management is often successfully used for acute patellar dislocations without the presence of a loose body. Occult subcortical OC fractures with an intact cartilage surface can usually be treated nonoperatively with protected weight bearing and restricted range of motion. Rarely a large subcortical depression fracture may warrant surgery. Arthroscopically assisted antegrade elevation with restoration of the normal joint surface curvature has been reported.[21]

Surgery is indicated in most cases of displaced OC fractures. Historically, OC fractures have been treated with excision and early range of motion.[15,16,18,31–33] Fixation of loose OC fragments was first described in the 1970s.[11] At present, fixation of weight-bearing condylar lesions is preferred unless the lesion is small or the OC fragment is damaged. If the loose OC fragment has minimal subchondral bone or a damaged chondral surface, or if the donor site is located in a non–weight-bearing area, loose body removal and donor site resurfacing are indicated. If the OC fragment is excised, options such as microfracture, OC autograft plugs, OC allografts, and ACI exist. Indications and techniques are described in the literature.[3,34–50] OC fractures with intact cartilage and sufficient subchondral bone that occur in the weight-bearing regions should be treated with reduction and fixation.[2] Several methods of fixation have been described in the literature.[2,12,17,19,23,51–58]

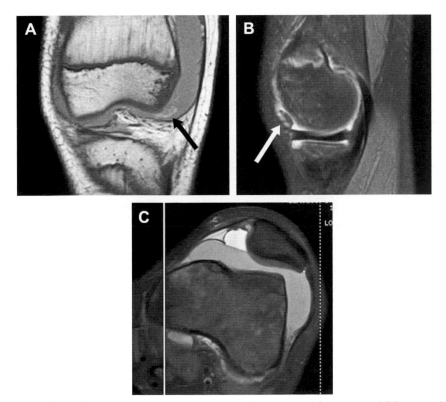

Fig. 2. Coronal T1 (*A*), sagittal proton density fat-saturated (*B*), and axial fat-saturated (*C*) magnetic resonance images of a patellar dislocation with loose body (*black arrow* on coronal, *white arrow* on sagittal).

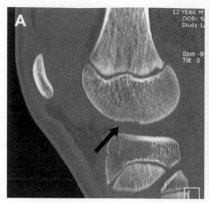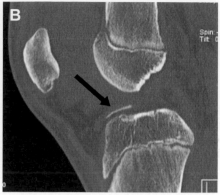

Fig. 3. Sagittal computed tomography scans following a traumatic knee injury in a 13-year-old patient. Note the donor site (*A*) and OC fracture fragment (*B*) (*black arrows*).

REDUCTION AND REPAIR OF OC FRACTURES
The Authors' Preferred Technique

Initial arthroscopic assessment followed by appropriate exposure and rigid fixation is the preferred technique. For patients with a loose OC fracture after an acute patellar dislocation, both injuries must be addressed. A standard knee arthroscopy is performed and the hemarthrosis is lavaged. The OC fragment is often discovered in the suprapatellar pouch. An accessory superolateral or superomedial portal can facilitate the removal of loose body, which should be done carefully to avoid damaging the chondral surface of the fragment. The loose body is then inspected to establish whether the fragment has sufficient subchondral bone attached and to examine the status of the overlying cartilage. The donor site is next evaluated to determine if it is in a weight-bearing articular area. For trochlear lesions, the knee should be flexed to find out if the donor site is located under the patella during normal motion.

For patellar and trochlear lesions, a mini-arthrotomy is usually required to best access the donor site for reduction and fixation. Lesions on the medial aspect of the patella in the setting of a patellar dislocation can often be accessed through the same incision used for an open medial retinacular repair that often accompanies this procedure.[58] Lesions on the lateral trochlea or lateral aspect of the patella may be accessed by a mini-lateral arthrotomy. A lateral retinacular release may facilitate patellar eversion and surgical exposure for lateral patellar lesions. An arthroscopic approach may be possible for lateral trochlear lesions. In these cases, an accessory superolateral portal is created directly over the area of repair to facilitate perpendicular access to the lesion.

Femoral condyle OC fractures are often best accessed with a mini-arthrotomy. The corresponding arthroscopic portal is extended in a longitudinal manner to access the lesion. If the lesion is far posterior, the knee can be hyperflexed for exposure.[58] For arthroscopic repair, a perpendicular path to the lesion must be established using an accessory portal, and the synovium should be cleared from the path. If multiple implants are thought to be necessary to achieve stable fixation, a mini-arthrotomy allows greater degrees of freedom for the fixation instruments and implants.

The donor site is first prepared by carefully removing the nonviable tissue from the donor base by using small curets. Excessive debridement is avoided to minimize the loss of bone and subsequent fragment depression. The chondral surface is then debrided to stable edges, and the subchondral bone is perforated to promote bleeding. If significant loss of subchondral bone exists, autologous bone graft may be packed into the donor site before reduction and fixation. The fragment is reduced and provisionally stabilized with 1 or 2 Kirschner wires. Depending on the length of time from injury, the fragment may need to be trimmed to facilitate reduction because of chondral swelling.

Definitive fixation is then performed (**Fig. 4**). The choice of implant depends on the preference and comfort level of the surgeon as well as the availability of implants. Fixation can be achieved with a variety of devices, including smooth or threaded pins, headless or low-profile compression screws (countersunk below the articular surface), bioabsorbable implants, and absorbable sutures. Partially threaded cannulated screws provide the most compression; however, they leave an indentation on the articular surface and, if not countersunk, may scuff the tibial surface, requiring later removal. Headless screws can be buried below the articular cartilage surface and provide compression, but

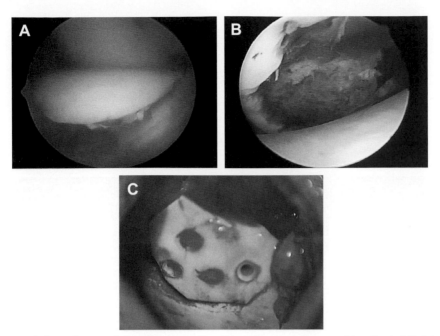

Fig. 4. Arthroscopic knee images following a patellar dislocation in a 15-year-old patient. (*A*) A loose body is identified and removed (note the subchondral bone on the loose fragment). (*B*) The donor site on the lateral femoral condyle (weight bearing) is identified and prepared. (*C*) The loose fragment is reduced and fixed into the donor site with bioabsorbable implants.

may back out over time and require removal. Bioabsorbable implants are useful for smaller lesions with scant subchondral bone, but are more costly and provide less interfragmentary compression in comparison with metallic devices.[34] Because of the lack of comparative studies or long-term follow-up studies in the pediatric population, no one implant can be recommended over another.

The authors' preference is to use bioabsorbable implants whenever possible to avoid the need for future implant removal. Examples of bioabsorbable implants include 1.5-mm or 2.4-mm bioabsorbablekl poly-(L-lactide) copolymer tacks (SmartNail, ConMed Linvatec, Utica, NY, USA) or a 2.7-mm bioabsorbable poly-(L-lactide) screw (Bio-Compression screw, Arthrex, Naples, FL, USA). The authors reserve metal screw fixation for very large unstable lesions in which significant compression is necessary to stimulate OC healing. Multiple fixation points are used for larger or more unstable lesions (**Fig. 5**). For smaller OC fragments, a single point of fixation through the center of the fragment or through the area of the fragment with the most subchondral bone attached is used. All fixation devices must be seated 1 to 2 mm below the level of the articular cartilage to prevent damage to adjacent weight-bearing areas.

For patellar lesions, shorter implants or even suture fixation may be necessary to avoid penetration of the dorsal cortex of the patella.[59] In the setting

of an OC fracture and patellar dislocation, a patellar stabilization procedure should be performed after OC fragment fixation. This often consists of an arthroscopic lateral retinacular release for patients with a tight lateral retinaculum followed by an open medial retinacular plication or repair.

Postoperative protocols vary after surgical treatment of acute OC fractures. For reduction and fixation of acute OC fractures, restricted knee range of motion may be instituted for the first 6 weeks depending on the location of the fracture site and other procedures performed. For patellofemoral lesions, full weight bearing may be allowed with the knee locked in full extension. When the patient is non–weight-bearing, the brace can be unlocked for passive range of motion exercises. The flexion angle of the knee at which the lesion makes patellofemoral contact is noted intraoperatively, and strength training is prevented at this degree of knee flexion for 4 months. For femoral condyle lesions, weight bearing is limited for 6 weeks postoperatively and impact sports activities are allowed after the healing of the lesion and the return of strength, which takes approximately 4 to 6 months.

RESULTS

Numerous reports detail that patellar dislocations often result in OC fractures.[7,10,28,60,61] However, sufficient data on reduction and fixation of acute

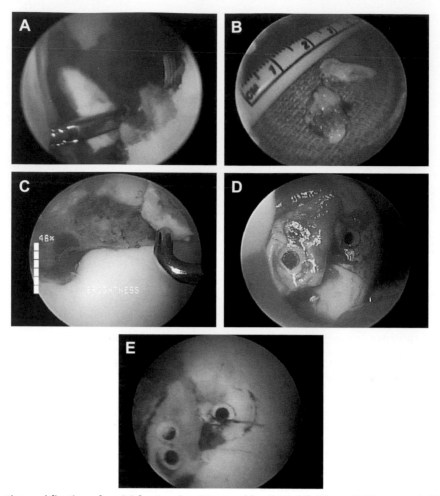

Fig. 5. Reduction and fixation of an OC fracture in a 16-year-old patient. (*A*) A loose OC fragment is identified and removed. (*B*) The fragments have subchondral bone attached. (*C*) The donor site is prepared. (*D*) The fragment is reduced and fixated through a mini-arthrotomy. (*E*) The reduced fragment is viewed during postfixation arthroscopy.

OC fractures are lacking. A few case reports detail operative technique and short-term outcomes.[59,62–64] Larger series with longer follow-up often include only a few patellar and trochlear lesions among the repair of OC fractures and osteochondritis dissecans lesions of the femoral condyles.[65,66] Most reports are case series that have, at most, a 2-year follow-up.[11,23,53,56,58] Walsh and colleagues[13] provided a 5- to 11-year follow-up on 8 patients (aged between 12 and 15 years) with large (>4 cm) LFC OC fractures that were treated with open reduction and internal fixation using bioabsorbable pins. The outcome of the treated knee was scored according to the International Knee Documentation Committee (IKDC) and Cincinnati Knee Rating systems. At final follow-up, 5 patients had an IKDC grade of A, 3 patients had a B grade, and 1 patient had a C grade. Five patients had no abnormalities on the knee radiographs, 2 patients had mild narrowing in the lateral compartment,

and 1 patient had mild femoral spurring. Evaluation by MRI showed all patients had intact articular surfaces, with only 1 patient showing a large area (2.8 × 4 cm) of abnormal and markedly thinned cartilage. This patient had an IKDC grade of A with no radiographic joint space narrowing at follow-up after 10 years.[13] Further research is indicated in this area.

MANAGEMENT OF POSTTRAUMATIC KNEE HEMARTHROSIS

Diagnosis of the traumatic knee abnormality in children can be difficult. Children often have difficulty remembering the exact mechanism of injury.[67] The physical examination in the injured child can also be challenging because of the patient's age, apprehension, and pain.[2] When the physical examination reveals a knee effusion after a traumatic injury, the effusion is most likely a hemarthrosis.[68] Radiographs are necessary and may identify physeal fractures and associated injuries but often miss smaller OC fractures.

Acute traumatic knee hemarthrosis in children often indicates underlying injury. One report of 44 consecutive patients with traumatic knee effusions found evidence for anterior cruciate ligament (ACL) tear in 29% of patients, meniscal tear in 29%, and OC fractures in 4%.[68] Stanitski and colleagues[69] noted ACL injury in 63% and meniscal injury in 46% in a series of 70 patients with knee hemarthrosis. OC fractures accounted for only 7% of the lesions. OC fractures may be more common especially in younger children. In another series of 21 consecutive children with open physes treated with knee arthroscopy, 14 of 21 (67%) children had an OC fracture of the patella or LFC.[6] Preoperative radiographs failed to identify the fracture in 5 (36%) of these 14 children.[6]

The difficulty in correctly diagnosing intra-articular knee pathology in children has been well documented.[6,70,71] Some investigators routinely recommend arthroscopy in the setting of a traumatic knee hemarthrosis in children.[70,72] However, this may lead to an invasive diagnostic modality in cases where surgery was unnecessary.[73,74] Although arthroscopy remains the gold standard, advances in MRI technique including gradient-echo sequences often allow for a noninvasive diagnosis and can aid surgical planning.[26,29,30] Some investigators have questioned the reliability of MRI to correctly diagnose knee pathology in children.[75–77] A prospective study on the value of knee MRI following hemarthrosis in children younger than 14 years found that MRI was able to make a diagnosis in all 29 patients who had no abnormalities on the radiographs.[78] All patients underwent subsequent arthroscopy: 3 chondral injuries were noted to be missed by MRI and 2 OC fractures were missed by both MRI and arthroscopy. The two missed OC fractures were diagnosed later during a subsequent arthrotomy for recurrent patellar instability. Retrospective review of the MRI's revealed the lesions, however the authors noted that gradient-echo sequences were not performed which made the diagnosis via MRI more difficult.[78] In cases of traumatic knee hemarthrosis where MRI does not show any abnormalities, diagnostic arthroscopy may be considered. The authors' preference in these cases is to initiate conservative management and reserve arthroscopy for persistent mechanical symptoms or effusion.

SUMMARY

Acute patellar dislocations may result in an OC fracture to the patella and/or trochlear groove.

Most cases of acute OC injuries to the pediatric knee result in hemarthrosis. The presence of a large hemarthrosis and loose body following a patellar dislocation is suggestive of an OC injury. OC injuries to the femoral condyles can also result from a direct blow to the knee, causing a shear injury. Large OC fragments on weight-bearing surfaces should be treated operatively with an attempt at repair if possible. Familiarity with the management of a posttraumatic knee hemarthrosis and operative techniques for repair of OC fractures is essential for the clinician and surgeon. Proper treatment can restore the native chondral surface. Further research is indicated to determine whether surgical repair in these cases prevents long-term disability from arthritis and to form evidence-based treatment algorithms.

REFERENCES

1. Flachsmann R, Broom ND, Hardy AE, et al. Why is the adolescent joint particularly susceptible to osteochondral shear fracture? Clin Orthop Relat Res 2000;(381):212–21.
2. Iobst C, Kocher M. Chondral injuries and osteochondral fractures. In: Micheli L, Kocher M, editors. The pediatric and adolescent knee. Philadelphia: Saunders; 2006. p. 294–316.
3. Micheli L, Curtis C, Shervin N. Articular cartilage repair in the adolescent athlete: is autologous chondrocyte implantation the answer? Clin J Sport Med 2006;16(6):465–70.
4. Peterson L, Minas T, Brittberg M, et al. Treatment of osteochondritis dissecans of the knee with autologous chondrocyte transplantation: results at two to ten years. J Bone Joint Surg Am 2003;85(Suppl 2): 17–24.
5. Birk GT, DeLee JC. Osteochondral injuries. Clinical findings. Clin Sports Med 2001;20(2):279–86.
6. Matelic TM, Aronsson DD, Boyd DW Jr, et al. Acute hemarthrosis of the knee in children. Am J Sports Med 1995;23(6):668–71.
7. Nietosvaara Y, Aalto K, Kallio PE. Acute patellar dislocation in children: incidence and associated osteochondral fractures. J Pediatr Orthop 1994; 14(4):513–5.
8. Stanitski CL, Paletta GA Jr. Articular cartilage injury with acute patellar dislocation in adolescents. Arthroscopic and radiographic correlation. Am J Sports Med 1998;26(1):52–5.
9. Costouros JG, Safran MR, Maletiz GB. Acute osteochondral defects in the knee. In: Mirzayan R, editor. Cartilage injury in the athlete. New York: Thieme Medical Publishers; 2006. p. 187–202.
10. Nomura E, Inoue M, Kurimura M. Chondral and osteochondral injuries associated with acute patellar dislocation. Arthroscopy 2003;19(7):717–21.

11. Matthewson MH, Dandy DJ. Osteochondral fractures of the lateral femoral condyle: a result of indirect violence to the knee. J Bone Joint Surg Br 1978;60(2):199–202.

12. Mashoof AA, Scholl MD, Lahav A, et al. Osteochondral injury to the mid-lateral weight-bearing portion of the lateral femoral condyle associated with patella dislocation. Arthroscopy 2005;21(2):228–32.

13. Walsh SJ, Boyle MJ, Morganti V. Large osteochondral fractures of the lateral femoral condyle in the adolescent: outcome of bioabsorbable pin fixation. J Bone Joint Surg Am 2008;90(7):1473–8.

14. Sanders TG, Paruchuri NB, Zlatkin MB. MRI of osteochondral defects of the lateral femoral condyle: incidence and pattern of injury after transient lateral dislocation of the patella. AJR Am J Roentgenol 2006;187(5):1332–7.

15. Becton JL, Linscheid RL. Osteochondral fracture of the medial femoral condyle: case report. Mayo Clin Proc 1966;41(4):242–5.

16. Coventry MB, Walt AJ. Osteochondral fracture of the femoral condyles. Surg Gynecol Obstet 1955; 100(5):591–4.

17. Gul R, Khan F, Maher Y, et al. Osteochondral fractures in the knee treated with butyl-2-cyanoacrylate glue. A case report. Acta Orthop Belg 2006;72(5):641–3.

18. Harmon PH. Intra-articular osteochondral fractures as a cause for internal derangement of the knee in adolscents. J Bone Joint Surg Am 1945;27(4):703–5.

19. Bowers AL, Huffman GR. Suture bridge fixation of a femoral condyle traumatic osteochondral defect. Clin Orthop Relat Res 2008;466(9):2276–81.

20. Vellet AD, Marks PH, Fowler PJ, et al. Occult posttraumatic osteochondral lesions of the knee: prevalence, classification, and short-term sequelae evaluated with MR imaging. Radiology 1991;178(1):271–6.

21. Gras F, Marintschev I, Koenig V, et al. Arthroscopic controlled reduction of femoral condyle fractures using a retrograde navigated approach. Arch Orthop Trauma Surg 2011;131(3):393–7.

22. Bellelli A, Nardis P. Occult or unknown traumatic osteochondral lesions of the knee. Assessment of 19 cases studied with conventional radiology and magnetic resonance. Radiol Med 1996;91(6):700–4 [in Italian].

23. Callewier A, Monsaert A, Lamraski G. Lateral femoral condyle osteochondral fracture combined to patellar dislocation: a case report. Orthop Traumatol Surg Res 2009;95(1):85–8.

24. Murray KJ. Hypermobility disorders in children and adolescents. Best practice & research. Clin Rheumatol 2006;20(2):329–51.

25. Capps GW, Hayes CW. Easily missed injuries around the knee. Radiographics 1994;14(6):1191–210.

26. Brittberg M, Winalski CS. Evaluation of cartilage injuries and repair. J Bone Joint Surg Am 2003; 85(Suppl 2):58–69.

27. Gomoll AH, Minas T, Farr J, et al. Treatment of chondral defects in the patellofemoral joint. J Knee Surg 2006;19(4):285–95.

28. Minas T. Surgical management of patellofemoral disease. In: Mirzayan R, editor. Cartilage injury in the athlete. New York: Thieme Medical Publishers; 2006. p. 273–85.

29. Potter HG, Foo LF. Magnetic resonance imaging of articular cartilage: trauma, degeneration, and repair. Am J Sports Med 2006;34(4):661–77.

30. Winalski CS, Gupta KB. Magnetic resonance imaging of focal articular cartilage lesions. Top Magn Reson Imaging 2003;14(2):131–44.

31. Makin M. Osteochondral fracture of the lateral femoral condyle. J Bone Joint Surg Am 1951;33(A:1):262–4.

32. Rosenberg NJ. Osteochondral fractures of the lateral femoral condyle. J Bone Joint Surg Am 1964;46: 1013–26.

33. Rorabeck CH, Bobechko WP. Acute dislocation of the patella with osteochondral fracture: a review of eighteen cases. J Bone Joint Surg Br 1976;58(2): 237–40.

34. Alford JW, Cole BJ. Cartilage restoration, part 2: techniques, outcomes, and future directions. Am J Sports Med 2005;33(3):443–60.

35. Azer N, Minas T. Treatment of articular cartilage lesions using autologous chondrocyte implantation. In: Micheli L, Kocher M, editors. The pediatric and adolescent knee. Philadelphia: Saunders; 2006. p. 303–7.

36. Bartlett W, Skinner JA, Gooding CR, et al. Autologous chondrocyte implantation versus matrix-induced autologous chondrocyte implantation for osteochondral defects of the knee: a prospective, randomised study. J Bone Joint Surg Br 2005; 87(5):640–5.

37. Bentley G, Biant LC, Carrington RW, et al. A prospective, randomised comparison of autologous chondrocyte implantation versus mosaicplasty for osteochondral defects in the knee. J Bone Joint Surg Br 2003;85(2):223–30.

38. Browne JE, Branch TP. Surgical alternatives for treatment of articular cartilage lesions. J Am Acad Orthop Surg 2000;8(3):180–9.

39. Bugbee WD. Fresh osteochondral allografts. J Knee Surg 2002;15(3):191–5.

40. Bugbee WD, Ostempowski MJ. Osteochondral allograft transplantation. In: Mirzayan R, editor. Cartilage injury in the athlete. New York: Thieme Medical Publishers; 2006. p. 158–69.

41. Chu CR, Convery FR, Akeson WH, et al. Articular cartilage transplantation. Clinical results in the knee. Clin Orthop Relat Res 1999;(360):159–68.

42. Erggelet C, Sittinger M, Lahm A. The arthroscopic implantation of autologous chondrocytes for the treatment of full-thickness cartilage defects of the knee joint. Arthroscopy 2003;19(1):108–10.

43. Frisbie DD, Oxford JT, Southwood L, et al. Early events in cartilage repair after subchondral bone microfracture. Clin Orthop Relat Res 2003;(407):215–27.

44. Hangody L, Fules P. Autologous osteochondral mosaicplasty for the treatment of full-thickness defects of weight-bearing joints: ten years of experimental and clinical experience. J Bone Joint Surg Am 2003;85(Suppl 2):25–32.

45. Jackson DW, Scheer MJ, Simon TM. Cartilage substitutes: overview of basic science and treatment options. J Am Acad Orthop Surg 2001;9(1): 37–52.

46. Kish G, Modis L, Hangody L. Osteochondral mosaicplasty for the treatment of focal chondral and osteochondral lesions of the knee and talus in the athlete. Rationale, indications, techniques, and results. Clin Sports Med 1999;18(1):45–66, vi.

47. Kreuz PC, Steinwachs MR, Erggelet C, et al. Results after microfracture of full-thickness chondral defects in different compartments in the knee. Osteoarthritis Cartilage 2006;14(11):1119–25.

48. Krishnan SP, Skinner JA, Bartlett W, et al. Who is the ideal candidate for autologous chondrocyte implantation? J Bone Joint Surg Br 2006;88(1):61–4.

49. Micheli LJ, Moseley JB, Anderson AF, et al. Articular cartilage defects of the distal femur in children and adolescents: treatment with autologous chondrocyte implantation. J Pediatr Orthop 2006;26(4):455–60.

50. Mithoefer K, Williams RJ 3rd, Warren RF, et al. The microfracture technique for the treatment of articular cartilage lesions in the knee. A prospective cohort study. J Bone Joint Surg Am 2005;87(9):1911–20.

51. Braune C, Rehart S, Kerschbaumer F, et al. Resorbable pin refixation of an osteochondral fracture of the lateral femoral condyle due to traumatic patellar dislocation: case management, follow-up and strategy in adolescents. Z Orthop Ihre Grenzgeb 2004;142(1):103–8 [in German].

52. Dines JS, Fealy S, Potter HG, et al. Outcomes of osteochondral lesions of the knee repaired with a bioabsorbable device. Arthroscopy 2008;24(1):62–8.

53. Jehan S, Loeffler MD, Pervez H. Osteochondral fracture of the lateral femoral condyle involving the entire weight bearing articular surface fixed with biodegradable screws. J Pak Med Assoc 2010;60(5):400–1.

54. Keller J, Andreassen TT, Joyce F, et al. Fixation of osteochondral fractures. Fibrin sealant tested in dogs. Acta Orthop Scand 1985;56(4):323–6.

55. Lewis PL, Foster BK. Herbert screw fixation of osteochondral fractures about the knee. Aust N Z J Surg 1990;60(7):511–3.

56. Lüthje P, Nurmi-Lüthje I. Osteochondral fracture of the knee treated with bioabsorbable implants in two adolescents. Acta Orthop Belg 2008;74(2):249–54.

57 Meyers MH, Herron M. A fibrin adhesive seal for the repair of osteochondral fracture fragments. Clin Orthop Relat Res 1984;(102):258–63

58. Taitsman LA, Frank JB, Mills WJ, et al. Osteochondral fracture of the distal lateral femoral condyle: a report of two cases. J Orthop Trauma 2006; 20(5):358–62.

59. Dhawan A, Hospodar PP. Suture fixation as a treatment for acute traumatic osteochondral lesions. Arthroscopy 1999;15(3):307–11.

60. Kramer D, Kocher M. Management of patellar and trochlear chondral injuries. Operat Tech Orthop 2007;17(4):234–43.

61. Luhmann SJ, Schoenecker PL, Dobbs MB, et al. Arthroscopic findings at the time of patellar realignment surgery in adolescents. J Pediatr Orthop 2007; 27(5):493–8.

62. Goh SK, Koh JS, Tan MH. Knee locking secondary to osteochondral fracture of the patella: an unusual presentation. Singapore Med J 2008;49(6):505–6.

63. Hoshino CM, Thomas BM. Late repair of an osteochondral fracture of the patella. Orthopedics 2010;270–3.

64. Tonin M, Said AM, Veselko M. Arthroscopic reduction and fixation of osteochondral fracture of the patellar ridge. Arthroscopy 2001;17(4):E15.

65. Adachi N, Deie M, Nakamae A, et al. Functional and radiographic outcome of stable juvenile osteochondritis dissecans of the knee treated with retroarticular drilling without bone grafting. Arthroscopy 2009; 25(2):145–52.

66. Wachowski MM, Floerkemeier T, Balcarek P, et al. Mid-term clinical and MRI results after refixation of osteochondral fractures with resorbable implants. Z Orthop Unfall 2011;149(1):61–7 [in German].

67. Butler JC, Andrews JR. The role of arthroscopic surgery in the evaluation of acute traumatic hemarthrosis of the knee. Clin Orthop Relat Res 1988;(228):150–2.

68. Luhmann SJ. Acute traumatic knee effusions in children and adolescents. J Pediatr Orthop 2003;23(2): 199–202.

69. Stanitski CL, Harvell JC, Fu F. Observations on acute knee hemarthrosis in children and adolescents. J Pediatr Orthop 1993;13(4):506–10.

70. Angel KR, Hall DJ. The role of arthroscopy in children and adolescents. Arthroscopy 1989;5(3):192–6.

71. Morrissy RT, Eubanks RG, Park JP, et al. Arthroscopy of the knee in children. Clin Orthop Relat Res 1982;(162):103–7.

72. Haus J, Refior HJ. The importance of arthroscopy in sports injuries in children and adolescents. Knee Surg Sports Traumatol Arthrosc 1993;1(1):34–8.

73. Eiskjaer S, Larsen ST, Schmidt MB. The significance of hemarthrosis of the knee in children. Arch Orthop Trauma Surg 1988;107(2):96–8.

74. Harilainen A, Myllynen P, Antila H, et al. The significance of arthroscopy and examination under anaesthesia in the diagnosis of fresh injury haemarthrosis of the knee joint. Injury 1988;19(1):21–4.

75. McDermott MJ, Bathgate B, Gillingham BL, et al. Correlation of MRI and arthroscopic diagnosis of knee pathology in children and adolescents. J Pediatr Orthop 1998;18(5):675–8.

76. Stanitski CL. Correlation of arthroscopic and clinical examinations with magnetic resonance imaging findings of injured knees in children and adolescents. Am J Sports Med 1998;26(1):2–6.

77. Stanitski CL. Use and abuse of knee MRI in assessment of pediatric knee intraarticular disorders. J Pediatr Orthop 2004;24(6):747–8.

78. Wessel LM, Scholz S, Rüsch M, et al. Hemarthrosis after trauma to the pediatric knee joint: what is the value of magnetic resonance imaging in the diagnostic algorithm? J Pediatr Orthop 2001;21(3): 338–42.

"One Step" Treatment of Juvenile Osteochondritis Dissecans in the Knee: Clinical Results and T2 Mapping Characterization

Francesca Vannini, MD, PhD[a],*, Milva Battaglia, MD[b],
Roberto Buda, MD[a], Marco Cavallo, MD[a],
Sandro Giannini, MD[a]

KEYWORDS

- Osteochondritis dissecans • Juvenile • Knee
- Bone marrow–derived cells transplantation
- One-step surgical technique

Osteochondritis dissecans (OCD) is a joint disorder with an increasingly common cause of knee pain and dysfunction among skeletally immature and young adult patients, especially those involved in competitive sports. Although the average age at presentation is between 10 and 20 years, OCD may occur in people of any age group. Men are more likely (two to three times) to develop OCD than women. In the knee joint, the posterolateral area of the medial femoral condyle is the most commonly involved site. OCD is characterized by an acquired, idiopathic lesion of subchondral bone with osseous reabsorption, collapse, and sequestrum formation that causes a spectrum of osteochondral lesions, from softening of the intact articular cartilage to a complete separation of osteochondral fragments and intra-articular loose bodies. An osteochondral fragment may be present in situ, partially or completely detached.[1,2]

Although the origin of OCD remains controversial, plausible causes include endocrine disorders, familiar predisposition, vascular insufficiency, articular epiphyseal ossification aberrations, and repetitive trauma.[3–6] Different classifications of OCD have been proposed basing on anatomic location, age of occurrence (juvenile and adult forms), joint pathology, and radiographic (scintigraphy and MRI) findings.[3–9] Specifically, it is important to distinguish knee OCDs in skeletally immature patient from skeletally mature, because the natural history of cartilage growth, development, and repair varies in these two populations, with worse prognosis in patients with closed distal femoral physes.

Typically, the clinical signs and symptoms of OCD include pain, joint locking, decreased range of motion, swelling, tenderness, joint stiffness, and loose bodies (cartilage or osteochondral) in

Level of Evidence: Level IV, case series.
The authors have no conflicts of interest to disclose.
[a] II Clinic of Orthopaedics and Traumatology, Rizzoli Orthopaedic Institute, Via G.C. Pupilli 1, Bologna 40136, Italy
[b] Department of Radiology, Rizzoli Orthopaedic Institute, Bologna, Italy
* Corresponding author.
E-mail address: France vannini@yahoo.it

the joint. Treatment strategies of OCD are intended to restore the normal functioning of the affected joint and to alleviate pain. Early diagnosis and treatment of OCD, when most lesions are stable, is important in young patients to minimize the risk of long-term disability and provide the patient with more treatment options. If left untreated, OCD increases the risk of the patient eventually developing osteoarthritis in the affected knee. Although the ideal treatment strategy for OCD is still controversial, the osteochondral lesion of children whose bones are still growing may heal spontaneously with a period of rest and support. In a compliant patient with an immature epiphysis and a stable lesion, the likelihood is approximately 50% that the lesion will heal within 10 to 18 months with nonoperative treatment.[3]

Failure of nonoperative treatment, usually after at least 3 to 6 months, is an indication for operative intervention.[10–12] Drilling, open/arthroscopic fixation, fragment excision, microfractures, osteochondral grafting (autograft or allograft), and autologous chondrocyte implantation (ACI) have been described as viable surgical procedures.[11,13–20] Among them, when fixation is not possible, osteochondral plug replacement procedures have the advantage of repairing osteochondral defects with viable autologous cartilage and bone, which have the capability to integrate with the adjacent native tissue. However, donor site pathology, discontinuity in the orientation of the cartilage plugs, and fibrocartilage in the gaps are disadvantages of autografts, whereas the idea of transplanting freshly obtained allograft provides the option of having a high-quality viable tissue.[21,22] Cartilage regeneration using ACI instead provides a continuous cartilage repair with no or minimal donor site pathology.[23] However, because ACI treatment requires two operative procedures with associated high costs, new methods of cartilage regeneration have been sought.

The ideal treatment strategy with an optimal surgical technique to repair the osteochondral lesions in patients with OCD is still controversial. Recently, a new one-step surgical procedure based on the transplantation of bone marrow–derived cells (BMDCs) was proposed for osteochondral repair in the ankle and knee, and subsequently, because of the satisfactory results obtained, has also been indicated for juvenile OCD.[24,25] The rationale of BMDC transplantation is based on the capability of the multipotent cells along with their microenvironment to differentiate and regenerate both the cartilaginous and subchondral bone layer.[26–32]

The goal of this study was to evaluate and report the clinical and MRI findings for the treatment of OCD lesion of the knee with BMDC transplantation using a one-step surgical technique in six juvenile patients with a 3-year follow-up.

MATERIALS AND METHODS

The study protocol was approved by an independent ethical committee, and signed informed consent for participation in this investigation was obtained from all included patients.

PATIENTS

Six juvenile patients with OCD (four women and two men; mean age, 16 years; age range, 14–18 years) received osteochondral repair treatment in the affected knee with BMDC transplantation using a one-step surgical technique. Patients inclusion criteria were nonresponsiveness to conservative therapy and stage three to four osteochondral lesion, based on the International Cartilage Repair Society (ICRS) classification.[9] The mean osteochondral defect size of these patients was 4.6 ± 1.5 cm^3.

CLINICAL EVALUATION

To determine the clinical outcome, the knees were examined preoperatively and at 3 years' follow-up and evaluated using International Knee Documentation Committee (IKDC) scores. This scoring system provides a measure of function so that higher the scores reflect higher level of function and lower level of symptoms. According to this system, the lowest possible score is 18 and the highest possible score is 100. Therefore, a score of 100 indicates no limitation with daily living or sports activities, along with absence of symptoms.

MRI EVALUATION

Based on the protocol suggested by the ICRS,[9] MRI evaluation of the treated knee was performed at 3 years' follow-up in all cases using a three-dimensional Magnetic Resonance Observation of Cartilage Repair Tissue (MOCART) scoring system.[33] The MOCART criteria used to evaluate the cartilage repair were the (1) degree of filling of osteochondral defect (complete, hypertrophic, incomplete [inferior or superior to the 50% of the defect], exposure of subchondral bone); (2) integration of the regenerated tissue to the adjacent native tissue at the border zone (complete, incomplete); (3) surface of the regenerated tissue (intact, damaged inferior or superior to the 50% of the surface regenerated); (4) delayed-phase fast spin-echo (DPFSE) fat-saturated MR signal intensity of the regenerated tissue (isointense, moderately hyperintense, markedly hyperintense); (5)

integrity of the lamina and subchondral bone; and (6) presence of joint effusion and subchondral edema. Both depth (mm) and volume of the regenerated defect (mm^3) were calculated with manual trace. The volume was calculated with the formula of the ellipsoid (A × B × C × 4/3π).

MR images were obtained using a 1.5T MR scanner (Signa HDxt, GE Healthcare, Buckinghamshire, UK) and a dedicated phased array coil. DPFSE MR pulse sequence was used to obtain coronal (with and without fat saturation) and sagittal (with fat saturation) high-resolution images. For all the patients, MRI acquisition protocol at 3 years' follow-up was completed by coronal and sagittal T2 mapping high-resolution sequence with the following MR parameters: repetition time, 1000 ms; echo time range, 10 to 80 ms (for study of hyaline cartilage); matrix, 256 × 256; gap spacing 0; slice thickness 2 mm; and acquisition 1. T2 mapping was obtained using a multiecho (8 echoes train) and multislice (18 slices) sequence, with a total of 144 images acquired. Specific postprocessing T2 map software with final T2 grading-color maps had to be used for normal and regenerated cartilage. Coronal and sagittal MRI views were considered for T2 mapping evaluation. Measurement of the spatial distribution of the T2 map reveals areas with increased or decreased water content. These areas were measured with manual trace for single acquired slices.

In agreement with the study by Welsch and colleagues,[34] the regions of interest (ROIs) covering a cartilage repair tissue were positioned within the identified cartilage repair sites. In all cases, cartilage repair sites were seen on three to five contiguous sagittal and coronal sections, and two to three ROIs were placed within the regenerated tissue per section. A region of morphologically normal-appearing cartilage within the same knee was selected as a reference (control), with three ROIs positioned along the control cartilage tissue. Anatomically, because all areas of cartilage repair were located within the weight-bearing zone of the femoral condyle, and therefore the reference cartilage sites were also selected from the weight-bearing area of the femoral articular surface. Cartilage was defined as *normal* when full thickness was preserved relative to the adjacent native cartilage and the articular surface was intact, and if no intra-articular MR signal intensity variations were visible.

STATISTICAL ANALYSIS

All continuous data were expressed in terms of mean and standard deviation of the mean. A paired *t*-test was performed to test differences between basal and final measures, and MR T2

map value comparison between regenerated tissue and adjacent native cartilage (control). The Mann-Whitney test, evaluated using the Monte Carlo method for small samples, was performed to test differences between means of different groups. Spearman rank correlation was performed to investigate the relationships between continuous variables. For all tests, a *P* value less than 0.05 was considered significant. Because of the small sample, the authors decided to report all the Spearman correlations greater than 0.6. Statistical analysis was performed using the Statistical Package for the Social Sciences (SPSS) software version 15.0 (SPSS Inc., Chicago, Illinois, USA).

SURGICAL TECHNIQUE
Platelet Gel Production

A total of 120 mL of the patient's venous blood was obtained and processed the day before surgery with the Vivostat System (Vivolution, Denmark, Birkeroed) to provide 6 mL of platelet-rich fibrin (PRF) gel.[21]

Bone Marrow Aspiration

With the patient prone under spinal or general anesthesia, a total of 60 mL bone marrow aspirate was harvested from the posterior iliac crest with a marrow needle (size, 11 gauge × 100 mm) inserted 3 cm deep into the iliac bone. An aliquote of 5-mL bone marrow was aspirated from the iliac crest into a 20 mL plastic syringe internally coated with calcium–heparin solution. This procedure was repeated several times through the same skin opening until a total of 60 mL of bone marrow aspirate was collected. The marrow was aspirated in small fractions from different points to maximize the harvesting of the marrow stromal cells and to reduce dilution by peripheral blood.

Bone Marrow Concentration

The harvested bone marrow was processed directly in the operating room through removing most of the erythrocytes and plasma. A cell separator (Smart PReP, Harvest Technologies Corp., Plymouth, MA, USA) consisting of a centrifuge and a disposable double chamber device, provided 6 mL of concentrate containing nucleated cells after 15 minutes of multiple centrifugation cycles.

Arthroscopic BMDC Transplantation

After the bone marrow harvesting phase, a standard knee arthroscopy was performed, with the patient in the supine position. The OCD lesion was identified (**Fig. 1**), and the detached fragment was removed and measured (**Fig. 2**). A flipped

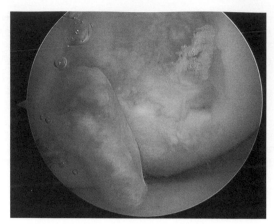

Fig. 1. Arthroscopic view of an OCD lesion showing the detached and dislocated fragment.

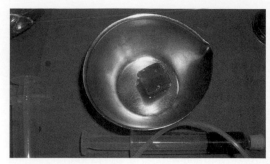

Fig. 3. The HA scaffold was loaded with 2 mL of bone marrow concentrate.

cannula was inserted into the portal ipsilateral to the lesion to enable insertion of the surgical instrumentations and to retract the fat pad from the operative field.[14] Using a specifically designed low-profile drill, the debridement of the osteochondral lesion was performed to create a circular biomaterial implantation site area with surrounding healthy native cartilage margins.

A hyaluronic acid (HA) membrane (Hyalofast, Fidia Advanced Biopolymers, Abano Terme, Italy) was used for cell support. The scaffold was filled with 2 mL of bone marrow concentrate (Fig. 3), and loaded onto the delivery device, which was used to position the biomaterial within the defect. Multiple stamp-sized pieces of HA membrane were overlapped to fill the osteochondral defect volume (Fig. 4). A layer of PRF gel was finally applied onto the implanted material to provide growth factors for osteochondral repair. Using carefully

controlled arthroscopy, the stability of the implanted osteochondral stamps was evaluated.

Postoperative Rehabilitation Program

Postsurgical rehabilitation involved a period of non–weight-bearing, during which the patients were encouraged to have gradual passive mobilization of the operated knee. Four weeks after the surgery the rehabilitation program included muscular reinforcement exercises, closed kinetic chain proprioceptive rehabilitation, swimming, and static and walking exercises progressing from partial to gradual weight-bearing. Ten weeks after the surgery the patients were allowed open kinetic chain rehabilitation exercises for the recovery of muscular function, and cycling and walking with full weight-bearing. After 6 months postsurgery, the patients were permitted light running, and after 12 months the patients could be involved with high-impact sports. The goal of this rehabilitation program for the patients was to

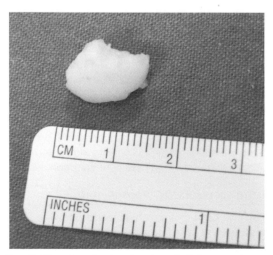

Fig. 2. The detached osteochondral fragment was measured.

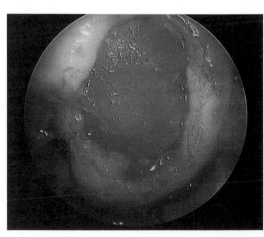

Fig. 4. The biomaterial (consisting of HA scaffold with 2 mL of bone marrow concentrate) was arthroscopically positioned onto the lesion site and multiple stamps were overlapped to cover the entire osteochondral defect area.

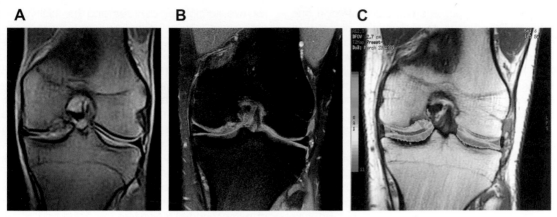

Fig. 5. Fifteen-year-old boy. (*A*) Preoperative coronal DPFSE MR image shows an OCD lesion of the medial femoral condyle. The preoperative clinical score was 68. (*B*) At 3 years' follow-up, sagittal DPFSE fat-saturated MR image showing complete defect filling, complete integration to border zone, and surface integrity of the regenerated tissue. Minimal subchondral bone edema is noted. (*C*) MRI T2 mapping shows regenerated tissue signal with a mean values of 40 ± 8 ms with respect to tissue control signal value of 28 ± 8. A focal area of higher water content is evident within the regenerated tissue. IKDC subjective score was 95.

ensure gradual progression from a period of non–weight-bearing and extensive physical therapy (to regain range of motion, strength, flexibility, and coordination) to full weight-bearing.

RESULTS
Clinical

No intraoperative or postoperative severe adverse events were reported in the patient cohort for this study. IKDC subjective showed a general improvement from 61.0 ± 4.5 preoperative to 96.5 ± 3.1 at the latest follow-up of 3 years

(*P*<.0005), indicating that overall the patients were able to resume most daily living and sports activities with significant reduction of symptoms. All patients declared that they were satisfied with the treatment. A negative influence of the size of the lesion on the percentage of improvement of the clinical score was seen (Rho = 0.618; *P* = .19).

MRI Scoring

MRI results evaluated using MOCART score[33] in DPFSE fat-saturated MR images showed a complete defect filling in four patients and hypertrophic in two patients. Integration to border zone was

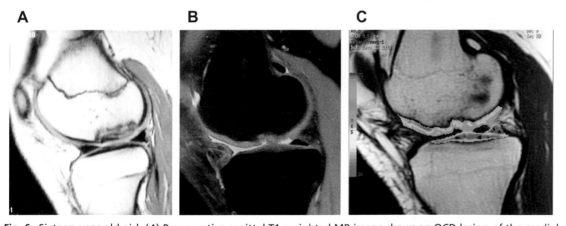

Fig. 6. Sixteen-year-old girl. (*A*) Preoperative sagittal T1-weighted MR image shows an OCD lesion of the medial femoral condyle with the fragment in situ. The preoperative clinical score was 58. (*B*) At 3 years' follow-up, sagittal DPSE fat-saturated MR image showing complete defect filling, integration to border zone, surface integrity of regenerated tissue with a focal damage. Subchondral edema was not seen. Compared with the preoperative MR image (*A*), a morphologically good OCD defect filling with regenerated cartilage and bone was noted. (*C*) T2 map shows MR signal of regenerated tissue with a mean T2 value of 45 ± 7 ms compared with the control MR signal with T2 value of 36 ± 8. The higher water content of regenerated tissue could indicate the cartilaginous remodeling phase. IKDC subjective score was 100.

complete in five patients and incomplete in one patient. The surface of regenerated tissue was intact (type 3) in five patients and damaged (type 1) in one patient. The reparative tissue was moderately hyperintense (type 2) and the subchondral lamina was damaged in all patients. Joint effusion was never evident, although two patients had subchondral edema.

When the degree of filling of osteochondral defect resulted complete, this had a tendency to positively impact both the clinical score (defect with a complete filling resulted in 98 ± 2.4 points, compared with evidence of hypertrophic tissue of 93 ± 2 points; $P = .09$) and the percentage of clinical improvement (94% ± 7% compared with evidence of hypertrophic tissue of 83% ± 4%; $P = .12$). Furthermore, when comparing MRI before treatment and at 3-year follow-up, subchondral bone regeneration was evident in all cases. No correlations were seen between the remaining MOCART parameters and the clinical score.

MRI T2 Mapping

The T2 map value of the regenerated tissue (43.5 ± 3 ms) was significantly higher ($P<.0005$) with respect to the healthy cartilage control (32 ± 3 ms). Otherwise, no tendency for a positive impact on the clinical score was correlated with regenerated tissue with a T2 map value closer to the control. Instead, a T2 map value with higher water content (compatible with a tissue in remodeling phase) was found to have a positive impact both on the final clinical score (Rho = 0.618; $P = .19$) and on the percentage of improvement obtained (Rho = 0.627; $P = .18$). No correlations were found on the other T2 map parameters and the clinical score.

DISCUSSION

This study investigated the clinical outcome of a recently developed one-step surgical approach for treating juvenile OCD of the knee with BMDC transplantation. The average follow-up in this study was 3 years. In general, it is desirable to fix the loose osteochondral fragment. However, eventually the osteochondral fragment cannot be preserved, or it fails to heal after initial fixation.[13,32]

Different techniques have been proposed over time for OCD treatment, and particularly ACI technique, introduced in 1994 by Brittberg and colleagues,[23] has proven to regenerate cartilaginous tissue with biomechanical properties comparable to those of the surrounding healthy cartilage, and is biomechanically superior to regenerated cartilage induced by other techniques.[14] Still, the need

for two surgical procedures and the high costs associated with cell expansion have been major drawbacks of ACI, which led to the search for new methods for cartilage repair.

The rationale of the one-step technique is based on the idea to transplant the entire bone marrow cellular pool instead of isolated and expanded mesenchymal stem cells.[24] This technique allows cells to be processed directly in the operating room, without the need for a laboratory phase, and enables BMDC transplantation to be performed using the one-step instead of the two-steps technique required for ACI.[31,32] The one-step surgery was previously used in the treatment of osteochondral lesions of the ankle and of the knee, resulting in satisfactory outcomes.[24,25] Buda and colleagues[25] reported a series of 20 patients affected by osteochondral lesion of the knee who underwent surgery using the arthroscopic one-step procedure. The mean IKDC score before surgery was 32.9 ± 14.2, and at 29 ± 4.1 months' postsurgery it was 90.4 ± 9.2 ($P<.0005$). The Knee Injury and Osteoarthritis Outcome Score (KOOS) before surgery was 47.1 ± 14.9, and at 29 ± 4.1 months' postsurgery it was 93.3 ± 6.8 ($P<.0005$). The clinical improvement was statistically significant both for IKDC and KOOS scores at each follow-up, with clinical improvement over time. The control MRI showed a good regeneration of the lesion site in different parameters of the MOCART score.

Mesenchymal stem cells, representing 2% to 3% of the total mononuclear cells in the bone marrow, have the ability to differentiate into various lineages, including osteoblasts and chondroblasts.[26,32] Biopsies of regenerated tissues revealed cartilaginous features, including a high expression of the major macromolecular components of articular cartilage, namely collagen type II and proteoglycans. When choosing a surgical management for OCD, particularly in juvenile OCD because of the young age of the patients, obtaining a repair tissue with cartilaginous features as close as possible to hyaline cartilage is essential. The treatment strategy for OCD lesions used in the patient cohort was aimed at treating both cartilage and subchondral bone lesions. The authors were able to obtain satisfactory clinical results in the treatment of a series of six juvenile patients with OCD in a single-step surgery. All patients showed a reduction in symptoms, increase in function, and stability of results over time.

A second-look biopsy of the regenerated tissue is invasive and unjustified in an asymptomatic knee; furthermore, it provides only information regarding a small portion of the regenerated area. On the contrary, a standard MRI can provide important morphologic information, such as percentage of filling defects, surface integrity of regenerated tissue, and the integration of the regenerated tissue with the surrounding native tissue. Although an MRI cannot be used to directly evaluate the regenerated tissue, recent advances in the MRI technology have improved the capability to provide information about the biochemical or molecular composition of regenerated tissue. An advanced MRI T2 mapping sequence provides supplemental information about the extracellular matrix of reparative tissue and, for this reason, it was used in this study to evaluate the quality of the regenerated tissue.[35–37]

In this study, all patients were evaluated using MOCART score and T2 mapping. The regenerated tissue filled the whole volume of the osteochondral lesions in all the cases. Five cases showed regenerated tissue with an intact surface, which integrated well with the surroundings native cartilage. Only in one case the regenerated tissue showed an irregular surface with damage inferior to 50% of the regenerated tissue. Nevertheless, this patient obtained a full clinical score. In two patients, subchondral edema was also present. Although Alparslan and colleagues[38] reported that presence of subchondral edema had an influence on the clinical score, in this study the presence of subchondral edema in the couple of patients did not have an impact on the clinical score. Furthermore, this series showed that BMDC transplantation had the capability to regenerate a large amount of subchondral bone, even if the defect was not filled by cancellous bone intraoperatively. These data are not in accord with a previous report describing the results of BMDC transplantation in the ankle joint, wherein the capability to regenerate subchondral bone along with cartilage seemed insufficient.[39] The outcome of these data may have been so positive because of the location of the defect or the younger age of the patients in this study.

T2 mapping was capable of detecting regenerated tissue, with T2 values higher with respect to healthy hyaline cartilage areas used for control (**Figs. 5C** and **6C**). Nevertheless, the presence of this tissue with higher water content, possibly referring to cartilage in the remodeling phase, was found to have a positive impact on the final clinical score and on the degree of improvement noted. However, no tendency to positively impact the clinical score was correlated with regenerative tissue with a T2 map value closer to the control. Interpretation of these data is difficult, and may be related to the small size of the sample. However, a previous study showed that the tissue with higher water content, considered as cartilage still in the remodeling phase, did not have a negative impact on the clinical score. On the opposite,

the presence of tissue with lower water content (fibrocartilage) negatively affected the clinical outcome.[39]

This study showed that the OCD treatment strategy of transplanting bone marrow–derived mesenchymal cells can provide good clinical and MRI (qualitative and quantitative) results. The treatment strategy used in this series had the goal of treating both cartilage and subchondral bone and provided satisfactory clinical results in the treatment of OCD in a single-step surgery. Patients showed a reduction in symptoms, increase in function, and stability of the results over time. MRI showed a satisfactory morphologic repair of the defect, whereas T2 mapping showed a reparative tissue with higher water content relative to healthy cartilage, which implies cartilage that is still in the remodeling phase. The limitations of this study include the small number of patients and relatively short follow-up. Further clinical and MRI follow-up are required to check the evolution of the reparative tissue obtained with the one-step procedure for the treatment of juvenile OCD in the knee and to determine whether cartilage will further progress toward hyaline features.

REFERENCES

1. Crawford DC, Safran MR. Osteochondritis dissecans of the knee. J Am Acad Orthop Surg 2006; 14(2):90–100.
2. Kocher MS, Tucker R, Ganley TJ, et al. Management of osteochondritis dissecans of the knee: current concepts review. Am J Sports Med 2006;34:1181–91.
3. Cahill BR. Osteochondritis dissecans of the knee: treatment of juvenile and adult forms. J Am Acad Orthop Surg 1995;3:237–47.
4. Clanton TO, DeLee JC. Osteochondritis dissecans: history, pathophysiology and current treatment concepts. Clin Orthop Relat Res 1982;167:50–64.
5. Glancy GL. Juvenile osteochondritis dissecans. Am J Knee Surg 1999;12:120–4.
6. Pappas A. Osteochondritis dissecans. Clin Orthop Relat Res 1981;158:59–69.
7. Cahill BR, Berg BC. 99m-technetium phosphate compound joint scintigraphy in the management of juvenile osteochondritis dissecans of the femoral condyles. Am J Sports Med 1983;11:329–35.
8. Hefti F, Beguiristain J, Krauspe R, et al. Osteochondritis dissecans: a multicenter study of the European Pediatric Orthopedic Society. J Pediatr Orthop B 1999;8:231–45.
9. Brittberg M, Winalski CS. Evaluation of cartilage injuries and repair. J Bone Joint Surg Am 2003;85:58–69.
10. Linden B. Osteochondritis dissecans of the femoral condyles: a long-term follow-up study. J Bone Joint Surg Am 1977;59:769–76.

11. Hughston JC, Hergenroeder PT, Courtenay BG. Osteochondritis dissecans of the femoral condyles. J Bone Joint Surg Am 1984;66:1340–8.

12. Van Demark R. Osteochondritis dissecans with spontaneous healing. J Bone Joint Surg Am 1952; 34:143–8.

13. Ramirez A, Abril JC, Chaparro M. Juvenile osteochondritis dissecans of the knee: perifocal sclerotic rim as a prognostic factor of healing. J Pediatr Orthop 2010;30(2):180–5.

14. Peterson L, Minas T, Brittberg M, et al. Treatment of osteochondritis dissecans of the knee with autologous chondrocyte transplantation: results at two to ten years. J Bone Joint Surg Am 2003;85(Suppl 2): 17–24.

15. Aglietti P, Buzzi R, Bassi PB, et al. Arthroscopic drilling in juvenile osteochondritis dissecans of the medial femoral condyle. Arthroscopy 1994;10:286–91.

16. Aichroth P. Osteochondritis dissecans of the knee: a clinical survey. J Bone Joint Surg Br 1971;53: 440–7.

17. Cahill B. Treatment of juvenile osteochondritis dissecans and osteochondritis dissecans of the knee. Clin Sports Med 1985;4:367–84.

18. Cain EL, Clancy WG. Treatment algorithm for osteochondral injuries of the knee. Clin Sports Med 2001; 20:321–42.

19. Kivisto R, Pasanen L, Leppilahti J, et al. Arthroscopic repair of osteochondritis dissecans of the femoral condyles with metal staple fixation: a report of 28 cases. Knee Surg Sports Traumatol Arthrosc 2002;10:305–9.

20. Donaldson LD, Wojtys EM. Extraarticular drilling for stable osteochondritis dissecans in the skeletally immature knee. J Pediatr Orthop 2008;28:831–5.

21. Hangody L, Ráthonyi GK, Duska Z, et al. Autologous osteochondral mosaicplasty. Surgical technique. J Bone Joint Surg Am 2004;86(Suppl 1):65–72.

22. Emmerson BC, Görtz S, Jamali AA, et al. Fresh osteochondral allografting in the treatment of osteochondritis dissecans of the femoral condyle. Am J Sports Med 2007;35(6):907–14.

23. Brittberg M, Lindahl A, Nilsson A, et al. Treatment of deep cartilage defects in the knee with autologous chondrocyte transplantation. N Engl J Med 1994; 331:889–95.

24. Giannini S, Buda R, Vannini F, et al. One-step bone marrow-derived cell transplantation in talar osteochondral lesions. Clin Orthop Relat Res 2009; 467(12):3307–20.

25. Buda R, Vannini F, Cavallo M, et al. Osteochondral lesions of the knee: a new one-step repair technique with bone-marrow-derived cells. J Bone Joint Surg Am 2010;92(Suppl 2):2–11.

26. Bosnakovski D, Mizuno M, Kim G, et al. Chondrogenic differentiation of bovine marrow mesenchymal stem cells (MSCs) in different hydrogels: influence of collagen type II extracellular matrix on MSC chondrogenesis. Biotechnol Bioeng 2006;93:1152–63.

27. Dominici M, Pritchard C, Garlits JE, et al. Hematopoietic cells and osteoblasts are derived from a common marrow progenitor after bone marrow transplantation. Proc Natl Acad Sci U S A 2004; 101:11761–6.

28. Kacena MA, Gundberg CM, Horowitz MC. A reciprocal regulatory interaction between megacaryocytes, bone cells and hematopoietic stem cells. Bone 2006;39: 978–84.

29. Longobardi L, O'Rear L, Aakula S, et al. Effect of IGF-I in the chondrogenesis of bone marrow mesenchymal stem cells in the presence or absence of TGF-beta signalling. J Bone Miner Res 2006;21: 626–36.

30. Lucarelli E, Beccheroni A, Donati D, et al. Platelet-derived growth factors enhance proliferation of human stromal stem cells. Biomaterials 2003;24: 3095–100.

31. Taichman RS. Blood and bone: two tissues whose fates are intertwined to create the hematopoietic stem-cell niche. Blood 2005;105:2631–9.

32. Capone C, Frigerio S, Fumagalli S, et al. Neurosphere-derived cells exert a neuroprotective action by changing the ischemic microenvironment. PLoS One 2007;2:e373.

33. Welsch GH, Zak L, Mamisch TC, et al. Three-dimensional magnetic resonance observation of cartilage repair tissue (MOCART) score assessed with an isotropic three-dimensional true fast imaging with steady-state precession sequence at 3.0 Tesla. Invest Radiol 2009;44(9):603–12.

34. Welsch GH, Mamisch TC, Domayer SE, et al. Cartilage T2 assessment at 3-T MR imaging: in vivo differentiation of normal hyaline cartilage from reparative tissue after two cartilage repair procedures–initial experience. Radiology 2008;247(1):154–61.

35. Choi YS, Potter HG, Chun TJ. MR imaging of cartilage repair in the knee and ankle. Radiographics 2008;28(4):1043–59.

36. Gold GE, McCauley TR, Gray ML, et al. What's new in cartilage? Radiographics 2003;23(5):1227–42.

37. Mosher TJ, Dardzinski BJ. Cartilage MRI T2 relaxation time mapping: overview and applications. Semin Musculoskelet Radiol 2004;8(4):355–68.

38. Alparslan L, Winalski CS, Boutin RD, et al. Postoperative magnetic resonance imaging of articular cartilage repair. Semin Musculoskelet Radiol 2001;5(4): 345–63.

39. Battaglia M, Rimondi E, Monti C, et al. Validity of T2 mapping in characterization of the regeneration tissue by BMDC transplantation in osteochondral lesions of the ankle. Eur J Radiol 2011;80(2): e132–9.

Clinical Relevance of Scaffolds for Cartilage Engineering

Thomas F. LaPorta, MD[a],*, Alexander Richter, MD, MS[b],
Nicholas A. Sgaglione, MD[c], Daniel A. Grande, PhD[d]

KEYWORDS

- Articular cartilage defects • Cartilage scaffolds
- Surgical cartilage repair • Tissue engineering

Articular cartilage is a highly organized tissue with complex biomechanical properties and substantial durability.[1] Hyaline cartilage is a highly specialized connective tissue, which permits smooth frictionless movement of joints and comprises chondrocytes embedded in an abundant extracellular matrix (ECM). The ECM is synthesized and secreted by the chondrocytes and consists predominantly of type II collagen, proteoglycans, and water, along with smaller amounts of other collagen types and noncollagenous proteins.[2] The biomechanical properties of articular cartilage are largely dependent on the composition and the integrity of its ECM.

Articular cartilage, because of its avascular nature, has limited capability for self-repair and regeneration.[3,4] Defects of articular cartilage are of 2 main categories, partial-thickness and full-thickness defects.[4] Partial-thickness defects, on the one hand, are limited to the cartilage only and have no access to bone marrow–derived stem cells. Therefore, a chondral injury that does not violate the subchondral bone lacks an inherent ability to heal spontaneously, and may gradually expand with time.[5] Full-thickness cartilage defects, on the other hand, have access to the bone marrow–derived stem cells of the subchondral bone and undergo some spontaneous healing, to a degree, through the formation of fibrocartilage.[6,7] Fibrocartilage

has inferior mechanical and biological properties compared with hyaline cartilage and can also gradually break down with time, resulting in permanent degradation of structure and function, ultimately leading to symptomatology and dysfunction.[4] However, the natural history of an isolated articular cartilage lesion is not completely understood, nor is it clinically predictable which lesions will become symptomatic. Nevertheless, these defects lead to substantial patient morbidity and may progress to diffuse osteoarthritis if not treated early.[8]

Articular cartilage injuries are common in the knee joint across all age groups, but are being 16–19,diagnosed and treated more frequently in young athletes. In studies of knee arthroscopies, articular cartilage lesions were observed in 66% of 993 knees (median patient age, 35 years), 63% of 31,516 knees (mean patient age, 43 years), and 60% of 25,124 knees (mean patient age, 39 years).[9–12] Patients with symptomatic cartilage lesions often report pain, swelling, joint locking, stiffness, and clicking.[9,13,14] Symptoms may cause significant functional impairment, often limiting one's ability to play sports, work, and perform activities of daily living.[15] Young patients with isolated focal chondral defects in the knee have considerable impairment of their quality of life, similar to that of patients requiring knee replacements for

[a] Department of Orthopaedics, Long Island Jewish Medical Center, Street 270–05 76th Avenue, New Hyde Park, NY 11040, USA
[b] Department of Orthopaedics, North-Shore Long Island Jewish Medical Center, Street 300 Community Drive, Manhasset, NY 11030, USA
[c] Department of Orthopaedics, North-Shore Long Island Jewish Medical Center, University Orthopaedic Associates, 611 Northern Boulevard, Suite 200, Great Neck, NY 11021, USA
[d] Department of Orthopaedics, Feinstein Institute for Medical Research, North-Shore Long Island Jewish Medical Center, Street 350 Community Drive, Manhasset, NY 11030, USA
* Corresponding author.
E-mail address: tlaporta@aecom.yu.edu

Orthop Clin N Am 43 (2012) 245 251
doi:10.1016/j.ocl.2012.02.002

the treatment of end-stage arthritis and worse than that of patients with chronic anterior cruciate ligament–deficient knees.[16] Adolescent patients may be particularly susceptible to osteochondral shearing injuries and osteochondral fractures. In a bovine model, adolescent cartilage failed at a lower shear stress in comparison with immature or adult cartilage, and also showed significantly reduced fracture toughness, requiring less energy to initiate and propagate a crack to a failure.[17]

Because articular cartilage has limited ability to repair or regenerate itself, several cartilage repair techniques have been used to relieve symptoms and functional limitations.[9] Current treatments for cartilage injury include, but are not limited to, debridement, chondroplasty, marrow stimulation techniques (ie, microfracture), bioabsorbable screw/pin fixation, osteochondral autografting/allografting, and cell-based therapies using cultured autologous chondrocytes.

NONOPERATIVE THERAPY

Conservative nonoperative therapy can also be used to treat symptomatic knee lesions and includes physiotherapy, weight reduction, systemic analgesics, intra-articular injections, and orthotic interventions.[4] Not all articular cartilage defects are symptomatic, so careful assessment of other potential causes of knee pain is also crucial. These modalities in combination help not only improve range of motion and potentially strengthen the limb but also decrease forces on the knee joint itself. Furthermore, a wide variety of analgesic and nonsteroidal anti-inflammatory drugs can be used, either alone or in combination, to aid in pain relief and improvement of function.

Nonoperative treatment methods focus on the management of chondral lesions, and a few predictably result in structural hyaline cartilage restoration.[18] Surgical management should be considered if the patient's symptoms are consistent with an underlying cartilage defect and adequate nonoperative management fails to provide acceptable pain relief or increase in function. Multiple studies indicate that treatment strategies for cartilage repair can be based primarily on the location and size of the defect, with age as a potential prognostigator.[19] Patients must understand that rehabilitation is essential, and a successful outcome may not always result on returning to sports or stressful activities.

NONREPARATIVE/NONRESTORATIVE PROCEDURES

There is a wide spectrum of various treatment approaches. Surgical procedures, which include debridement, chondral shaving, and joint lavage, can help minimize pain and improve mobility, but they do not restore the structure or function of the diseased cartilage.[20,21] These procedures can be performed independently or in combination with other techniques to promote enhanced integration of the newly formed repair tissue with the surrounding native cartilage.[21,22] However, limitations to these techniques include perimeter chondrocyte injury between healthy and damaged cartilage after the removal of the injured cartilage as well as the potential reduction in long-term beneficial outcomes.[23]

REPAIR/BONE MARROW–STIMULATING TECHNIQUES

Bone marrow stimulation techniques have been commonly used for treating small symptomatic lesions of the articular cartilage in the knee.[24] Reparative or bone marrow stimulation techniques aim at initiating bleeding from the subchondral bone by perforating the subchondral plate, which permits the migration of bone marrow stromal cells to the lesion along with "super" blood clot formation.[25,26] The pluripotent cells are able to differentiate into fibrochondrocytes, which contribute to fibrocartilage repair of the lesion and to some degree of hyaline-like cartilage tissue. However, the overall concentration of the marrow cellular elements can be less than predictable and also declines with age.[27,28] The formation of a stable and adhesive blood clot that maximally fills the chondral defect is important, and it has been correlated with the success of bone marrow stimulation procedures. In addition, creating a contained lesion and removing the calcified cartilage layer at the base of the lesion is critical to achieving a stable base for filling the defect with a clot and an optimal adhesion of the clot.[24]

The reparative fibrocartilage that results from the successful reparative procedures consists of types I, II, and III collagen in varying amounts.[29] The fibrocartilage does not resemble the surrounding hyaline cartilage and has less type II collagen. Although fibrocartilage has inferior mechanical properties and does not restore hyaline cartilage, the formation of this cartilage layer does cover the exposed underlying bone, subsequently helping to reduce pain and swelling.[19] Examples of marrow stimulation techniques include abrasion arthroplasty, subchondral drilling, microfracture chondroplasty, and spongialization.[30] Although various marrow stimulation techniques have been proved to produce excellent short-term clinical outcomes, the clinical durability of marrow-stimulated repair tissue has shown an objective and functional decline with long-term follow-up.[31–33]

With osteochondritis dissecans or larger osteochondral defects and fractures, repair may be attempted using bioabsorbable screws, rods, or pins. Data in the pediatric population are limited to case reports or small case series, but show promising results. Fixation of lateral femoral condyle lesions with poly-D-dioxanone pins,[34] poly lactide rods,[35] or poly-L-lactic acid screws[36] showed good bony union on magnetic resonance imaging (MRI)[35,36] and osteochondral reintegration on second-look arthroscopy.[34] The largest case series to date consists of 8 patients treated with polyglycolic acid (PGA) rod fixation showed good functional results with more than 5 years of follow-up.[37] On MRI there were no full-thickness defects, with 6 of the 8 patients showing no or a small area of cartilage thinning. Osteochondritis dissecans has also been treated with bioabsorbable fixation in several case series. One study of 13 patients explored arthroscopic fixation with polylactide screws and showed a significant improvement in function and return to sport in 12 of the 13 patients, with all patients rating their knee function as improved or much improved.[38] In another study using polylactic rods in 9 skeletally mature adolescent and young adult patients, 8 of the 9 patients achieved radiographically united knees, with 7 patients having good to excellent results.[39] Bioabsorbable pin resorption was studied in 59 patients with 175 polydioxanone pins using MRI.[40] At 24 months only 20% of pins were visible on MRI and, although at 6 months 32% of patients had focal defects present, at later time points this dropped to only 4%. Bioabsorbable fixation shows promising results functionally and on imaging in specific clinical situations, but warrants further study in larger trials.

RESTORATIVE TECHNIQUES

The treatment of the pathologic condition of articular cartilage of the knee has traditionally focused on realignment osteotomies and prosthetic replacement, particularly in older patients. For example, high tibial osteotomies and knee replacements aim to unload and replace the articular surfaces, respectively. More recent restorative techniques have focused on more biological approaches to resurfacing. At present, there has been a greater tendency to use biological approaches to treat cartilage lesions, especially in younger patients.[41] Biological approaches include osteochondral grafting (mosaicplasty/osteochondral autograft transplantation and osteochondral allograft transplantation) and

autologous chondrocyte transplantation/implantation (ACI), which have been clinically used to restore cartilage function and structure.[31] Restorative strategies have been developed to promote the healing of injured cartilage through the transfer or formation of tissue that resembles native hyaline cartilage.[19] Osteochondral autografting, mosaicplasty, and osteochondral allograft attempt to replace the cartilage defect with host or donor articular cartilage in a single stage, whereas ACI attempts to generate hyaline or hyaline-like cartilage in a 2-step surgical procedure (an arthroscopic procedure to harvest chondrocytes and an open procedure to reimplant cells).[31]

Michelli and colleagues[15] surveyed 32 adolescent patients who underwent ACI for articular cartilage defects. Twenty-eight of the patients reported an improvement in their overall condition score. Osteochondritis dissecans was treated using ACI and produced integrated repair tissue with successful clinical results in more than 90% of patients at 2 to 10 years of follow-up.[42] This trial included 7 patients younger than 18 years, but does not specifically address the success rate in the adolescent patients.

Like many of the aforementioned procedures attempted thus far, these restorative strategies have been fraught with their own limitations, concerns, and problems while attempting to relieve pain, restore function, and delay or halt the progression of osteoarthritis. Although osteochondral autologous transfer and mosaicplasty have yielded results showing improved function and decreased pain, especially in full-thickness defects measuring 1 to 5 cm^2,[43] there still exists the issues of donor site morbidity, technically demanding issues (optimum orientation of the graft to restore the contour of the femoral condyle),[44] and the ability of the cartilage plug to integrate with the adjacent normal cartilage.[45,46] Similarly, ACI, used clinically to treat focal cartilage defects,[47] has significant limitations. The technique requires a 2-staged surgical procedure, including harvesting and repair procedures, which can be challenging because it necessitates suturing the harvested periosteum to adjacent articular cartilage.[48] Even if one were to put aside the technical issues, biology would still limit the procedure. Questions arise as to whether the cells would produce ECM in the proper ratio of cells to matrix, whether the cells would have characteristics such as alignment and metabolism similar to those of the surrounding normal cartilage, and whether the collagen fibers would form and orient properly within the different layers of cartilage. Furthermore, the complications of periosteal hypertrophy and/or delamination, inadequate cell supply, donor site morbidity, and arthrofibrosis have been documented.[49]

Although many of the currently available surgical techniques have had documented improvement of joint function, relief of pain, and overall enhancement of their quality of life, no method has been viewed as overwhelmingly superior.[45,50] Surgical procedures have had limited success in restoring native articular tissue both in structure and biomechanical properties.[4,45,50] Despite the advancements and attempts at comparative assessments of these treatments, the lack of a consensus regarding an optimal treatment for the surgical repair of cartilage has contributed to the continued investigation of more advanced techniques using tissue engineering.[50,51]

TISSUE ENGINEERING/SCAFFOLDS

The lack of a consistent, superior, and reliable methodology to promote the repair of cartilage defects has resulted in a greater interest in tissue engineering.[52,53] The strategy includes use of a viable cell source, a stable scaffold, and bioactive molecules, such as growth factors and morphogens. The approach involves a combination of these 3 principles to facilitate the repair of native articular cartilage (**Fig. 1**).[50] The cells selected also must have the capacity to proliferate and produce matrix. The cells cannot achieve this independently because there is a need for chemotactic agents to direct the cells along the appropriate pathway of growth and

differentiation. The scaffold is essential to stabilize, anchor, and orient the cell construct.

There are certain characteristics that should be considered when specific scaffolds are designed. Safran and colleagues[48] cited a comprehensive list stating that ideal scaffolds should be biocompatible, noncytotoxic, biodegradable, permeable, able to support and hold cells, mechanically stable, reproducible, readily available, and versatile for both full-thickness and partial-thickness lesions. When evaluating scaffolds, biocompatibility and a noncytotoxic nature ensures that there is no local inflammatory response or disruption of the surrounding tissues, which could prevent the cells from proliferation. In addition, while the scaffold needs to be stable and mechanically sound to support the cells, it also needs to serve as only a temporary load-sharing matrix that can eventually be fully replaced by the ECM of the cells. After remodeling, the scaffold should aid in the development of tissue-engineered cartilage with biphasic properties similar to those of the native cartilage, with approximately 80% fluid-fluid phase (80% water and <1% electrolytes) and 20% solid phase (10%–15% collagen type II and 5%–10% proteoglycans).[4,7,54]

When expanded in a monolayer culture, chondrocytes start to lose their chondrogenic phenotype, but then regain their native phenotype

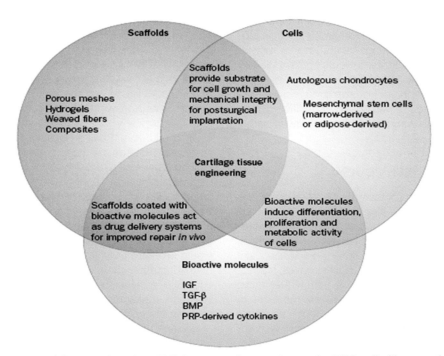

Fig. 1. Components of tissue engineering. BMP, bone morphogenetic protein; IGF, insulin-like growth factor; PRP, platelet-rich plasma; TGF, transforming growth factor. (*Data from* Daher RJ, Chahine NO, Greenberg AS, et al. New methods to diagnose and treat cartilage degeneration. Nat Rev Rheumatol 2009;5(11):599–607.)

when seeded in a 3-dimensional (3D) system using scaffolds.[45,55–57] Regarding versatility, the regenerated tissue derived from the cell/scaffold construct should entirely fill the defect in the native cartilage, regardless of size, and integrate optimally with the surrounding native cartilage.[48,58]

The scaffolds that have been described clinically thus far comprise a wide array of materials that include natural polymers, carbohydrates (hyaluronan, agarose, alginate, chitosan), and proteins (collagen, gelatin, fibrin), or synthetic/artificial polymers (polylactic acid [PLA], PGA, polyethylene oxide).[4,45,59] Many of these matrices are currently being tested, with much of the early attention being directed toward the natural polymers and more recent studies focusing on hybrids and synthetic scaffolds.

The ideal cell-carrier substance should be the one that closely mimics the natural environment in the cartilage-specific ECMs.[60] Carbohydrates, given the importance of glycosaminoglycans (GAGs) in stimulating chondrogenesis in vitro,[61,62] have been used as scaffolds to enhance the chondrogenesis required in the repair of chondral defects. Hyaluronan (also called hyaluronic acid [HA] or hyaluronate) is an anionic nonsulfated GAG that is widely distributed throughout connective, epithelial, and neural tissues. HA is a promising scaffold material used to promote cartilage repair and is important in tissue development, with elevated levels during early developmental phases (cellular proliferation and migration) and subsequent decreased levels as cells differentiate into mature phenotypes.[63] HA scaffolds have been shown to regulate, stabilize, and stimulate chondrogenesis. The HA scaffolds provide the structural support for cell contact and matrix deposition, but the 3D nonwoven HA scaffolds prevent dedifferentiation of chondrocytes as they bind to the HA through cell-surface receptors (CD44) and promote the expression of chondrocyte-specific markers, which induce signals that modulate cell proliferation, migration, and appropriate differentiation.[24] Previous studies of HA-based polymers in the repair of osteochondral defects has been associated with encouraging outcomes because the resulting tissue consisted of hyaline-like cartilage that appeared to be well integrated with the adjacent cartilage.[64] In addition, studies by Nettles and colleagues[65] in which HA was injected into a rabbit osteochondral defect model showed that HA integrated well with the native tissue, promoted the migration of cells, aided in the production of cartilage-specific matrix and, most importantly, served as a valuable scaffolding material.

Specifically, Hyalograft C (Fidia Advanced Biopolymers, Abano Terme, Italy) has received clinical attention. This HA-based scaffold is an esterified derivative of HA (ACP or HYAFF 11), which has been used alone and in combination with autologous chondrocytes that have been expanded in culture. Studies have shown that this scaffold supports the in vitro growth of chondrocytes and promotes the maintenance and expression of their original phenotype, with a decrease in the amount of type I collagen as well as an increase in the amount of type II collagen and *Sox9* production.[66,67] Hyalograft C has been investigated clinically with encouraging results, and histologic analysis has shown hyaline-like cartilage in the lesion as early as 12 months after implantation.[24] Marcacci and colleagues[68] conducted a multicenter clinical study with the primary objective of investigating the outcomes of patients treated with Hyalograft C. Clinical results of 141 patients, with follow-up assessments ranging from 2 to 5 years, were reported and showed that 91.5% of patients improved according to the International Knee Documentation Committee subjective evaluation, 76% had no pain, 88% had no mobility problems assessed by the EuroQol-EQ5D measure, and 96% had the involved knee rated as normal or nearly normal by the treating surgeon. Seventy patients of this group underwent biopsy of the lesion; at less than 18 months from implantation 46% had hyaline or mixed (hyaline and fibrous or fibrocartilage) cartilage, and at more than 18 months 69% had hyaline or mixed cartilage at the repair site.[48] Similarly, Gobbi and colleagues[69] looked at 32 patients with lesions, mainly in the patellofemoral region, treated with Hyalograft C. MRI studies were then conducted at 24 months and revealed that 71% of patients had almost normal cartilage with positive correlation to clinical outcomes, and 6 second-look arthroscopies revealed the repaired surface to be nearly normal with biopsy samples characterized as hyaline-like in appearance. These and several other studies, which have actually compared Hyalograft C with procedures such as ACI and microfracture, have shown that the use of this scaffold proves to be a more viable treatment of chondral lesions and achieves repair tissue associated with histologic characteristics similar to normal articular cartilage.[32,70,71]

More recently, other carbohydrates, including agarose, alginate, and chitosan, have gained attention. These substances have shown varying degrees of success for their potential to be incorporated either alone or in combination with other materials into scaffolds, and thus promote the production of components of a functional ECM, accumulate and attract cartilage markers, and maintain typical chondrocyte phenotype.[60,72–75]

Chitosan has been used extensively in a wide variety of scaffolds and different applications in articular cartilage tissue generation.[76] Specifically, a scaffold comprising chitosan and β-glycerophosphate, known as BST-CarGel, was introduced for clinical application by Biosyntech (Quebec, Canada). BST-CarGel was developed to stabilize the blood clot in the cartilage lesion by dispersing a soluble and adhesive polymer scaffold containing chitosan throughout uncoagulated whole blood.[77] Results in both animal studies and human trials have shown an increase in the volume and hyaline character of repair tissue, with increased GAG and collagen content especially when compared with microfracture controls.[78,79] Regarding clinical investigation, 33 human subjects were treated with BST-CarGel from August 2003 to December 2004 on a case-by-case basis involving a spectrum of both traumatic and degenerative lesions. The outcomes were monitored by Western Ontario McMaster (WOMAC) Osteoarthritis Index questionnaires administered preoperatively and again postoperatively after 3, 6, and 12 months.[77] Postoperatively at 12 months, WOMAC scores for pain, stiffness, and function improved significantly in patients treated with BST-CarGel, and although the results were recognized as anecdotal and short-term, the uniformity of the data suggested a clinical benefit following BST-CarGel treatment and has led to a current prospective, randomized, multicenter clinical trial in Canada comparing BST-CarGel with microfracture alone.[77]

Protein-based scaffolds have also experienced variable successes that have led to the approval of multiple carrier matrices and procedures across Europe and the United States for use in patients. These include collagen I/III-based scaffolds (Carticel, Chondro-Gide, Autologous matrix-induced chondrogenesis) and fibrin glue (FG) (Tissucol; Baxter, Deerfield, IL, USA); and the continued clinical investigation of many others involving collagen I/III (matrix-induced autologous chondrocyte implantation [MACI], Neocart, CaReS, Vericart), fibrin (DeNovo NT and ET grafts, Gelrin C), and gelatin. Collagen has been shown to display many of the ideal properties required for a scaffold, including high seeding efficiency, good cell adhesion, elasticity to conform to various shaped defects, preservation of cell viability and morphology, durability to tear, and elaboration of chondrocytic markers that all lead to more effective repair of osteochondral defects as they are filled with hyaline-like tissue.[4,80–83] In addition to the purely protein-based scaffolds are those scaffolds that involve a combination of natural polymers, such as Chondromimetic (Orthomimetics, Cambridge, UK), a novel biphasic biological scaffold comprising collagen and GAG.

Of the treatment methods using proteins as the scaffold, MACI (Genzyme Biosurgery, Cambridge, MA, USA) is one of the most widely used and clinically studied techniques, although it has not yet been released in the United States. This procedure is a modification of ACI and uses autogenous cells that are expanded in vitro, seeded between layers of a bilaminar collagen I/III scaffold (although other biomaterials have been used, ie, Hyalograft C),[9] and implanted into the defect with the construct held in place by an FG.[48] In multiple studies thus far, comparable results have been found between MACI and ACI procedures. Bartlett and colleagues[84] performed a prospective, randomized comparison of ACI-C (a modification of original ACI that uses porcine-derived type I/type III collagen as a cover) and MACI for the treatment of symptomatic chondral defects of the knee in 91 patients, of whom 44 received ACI-C and 47 MACI grafts, and after 1 year concluded that the clinical, arthroscopic, and histologic outcomes were comparable for both groups. Bartlett and colleagues[84] included adolescent patients as young as 15 years of age, but did not analyze these patients separately. Most recently, Zeifang and colleagues[85] randomized 21 patients with symptomatic, isolated, full-thickness cartilage defects at the femoral condyle to MACI or the original periosteal flap technique (ACI), with evaluation based on postoperative changes in knee function, quality of life, and physical activity at 3, 6, 12, and 24 months, and MRI at 6, 12, and 24 months to evaluate the repair of cartilage using the Magnetic Resonance Observation of Cartilage Repair Tissue score. At both 1 and 2 years after the procedure there was an improvement of patients' function, quality of life, activity level, and the Magnetic Resonance Observation of Cartilage Repair Tissue score following autologous chondrocyte implantation, but there was no significant difference between traditional ACI and MACI. Both of these examples illustrate that although MACI is technically appealing, further long-term studies are required before the technique becomes widely adopted.

Also in the protein family, commercial FG has long been used to secure tissue-engineered cartilage in clinical settings, and recently has been investigated and used clinically as a scaffolding material. Specifically, Denovo NT grafts (Zimmer, Warsaw, IN, USA; ISTO Technologies, St. Louis, MO, USA) showcase aseptically minced cartilage obtained from juvenile allograft donor joint, which creates a larger surface area for cartilage expansion, that is then is mixed intraoperatively with FG, which serves as a scaffold carrier allowing a chondroconductive milieu to be implanted into the lesion.[4,6]

Synthetic or artificial biodegradable scaffolds are currently undergoing different phases of early clinical investigation. These include scaffolds made from PGA (BioSeed-C, CAIS scaffolds), PLA (BioSeed-C), Polylactic coglycolic acid (TruFit bone substitute plus, BioSeed-C), and polyethylene glycol (Gelrin C, ChonDux). This class of scaffolds is interesting because they possess some of the important characteristics needed to function as an ideal scaffold, such as a high mechanical strength, a predictable degradation rate, high reproducibility, maintenance of chondrocyte morphology, promotion of the formation of an ECM resembling normal cartilage, and easy manipulation.[4,86,87]

One particular synthetic scaffold that has gained significant attention as a promising device for the treatment of osteochondral defects is the TruFit plug (Smith & Nephew, Andover, MA, USA), a synthetic resorbable biphasic implant. The device is made predominantly from PGA and poly-D,L-lactide-coglycolide fibers, which are preferentially aligned to provide good structure and are separated by appropriately sized pores, to allow ingrowth.[88,89] In addition, calcium sulfate forms 10% of the structure in its base, as well as a trace amount of surfactant.[88] The bilayer design of TruFit provides cartilage and bone phases yielding comparable mechanical properties for adjacent tissue. The implant is designed to fully resorb over time, potentially allowing for the complete filling of the defect with repair tissue to the same height as that of the surrounding articular surface.[90] Preclinical studies performed on osteochondral defects involving the medial femoral condyles and the distal-medial portion of the patellar grooves in goat models led to qualitative evaluations that showed repair sites with a high percentage of hyaline cartilage, good bony restoration, and the good integration of new tissue with the native cartilage.[91] These studies led to the clinical investigation of TruFit, which is approved in Europe for the treatment of acute osteochondral defects and by the US Food and Drug Administration only for backfill of osteochondral autograft sites.[92] Clinical investigation with the use of these plugs to repair cartilage in knees has thus far led to some conflicting clinical outcomes.[88,93–95] Most recently, Dhollander and colleagues[93] reported on 20 patients who were consecutively treated for their cartilage lesions with the plug technique. These patients were then prospectively clinically evaluated at 6 and 12 months of follow-up and also examined by MRI. The investigators noted the short-term clinical and MRI outcomes to be modest. Of the 15 patients followed up during 1 year, 3 were considered failures (20%) because they showed persistent clinical

symptoms or even more clinical symptoms after insertion of the plug.[93] These patients underwent revision surgery, and the histologic assessment of biopsy specimens taken showed fibrous vascularized repair tissue with the presence of foreign-body giant cells.[93]

SUMMARY

The treatment of cartilage defects represents a complex clinical challenge for orthopedic surgeons treating young and active patients. The few studies addressing cartilage defects in adolescents are relatively small scale. No one method has been viewed to be superior, and there remains a persistent lack of consensus regarding an optimal treatment. Some of the limitations of treatments have included an unpredictable tissue repair healing response, loss of transplanted tissues and cells, insufficient cell dedifferentiation, matrix destruction, and failure of integration between the subchondral bone in the defect and the regenerative tissue. These issues have led to a new generation of tissue-engineering techniques, which look to answer the questions of old and create potential repair strategies for cartilage defects. Through tissue engineering of cartilage, with its use of cells from various sources seeded on scaffolds made of various biomaterials, clinical advances may be realized in the regeneration of articular cartilage.

REFERENCES

1. Simon TM, Jackson DW. Articular cartilage: injury pathways and treatment options. Sports Med Arthrosc 2006;14:146–54.
2. Mankin HJ. The response of articular cartilage to mechanical injury. J Bone Joint Surg Am 1982; 64(3):460–6.
3. Marlovits S, Zeller P, Singer P, et al. Cartilage repair: generations of autologous chondrocyte transplantation. Eur J Radiol 2006;57:24–31.
4. Ahmed TA, Hincke MT. Strategies for articular cartilage lesion repair and functional restoration. Tissue Eng Part B Rev 2010;16(3):305–29.
5. Buckwalter J, Mankin H. Articular cartilage. Part II: degeneration and osteoarthrosis, repair, regeneration, and transplantation. J Bone Joint Surg Am 1997;79:612–32.
6. McCormick F, Yanke A, Provencher MT, et al. Minced articular cartilage—basic science, surgical technique, and clinical application. Sports Med Arthrosc 2008;16(4):217–20.
7. Temenoff JS, Mikos AG. Review: tissue engineering for regeneration of articular cartilage. Biomaterials 2000;21(5):431–40.

8. Alford JW, Cole BJ. Cartilage restoration, Part I: basic science, historical, perspective, patient evaluation, and treatment options. Am J Sports Med 2005; 33:295–306.

9. Brittberg M. Cell carriers as the next generation of cell therapy for cartilage repair: a review of the matrix-induced autologous chondrocyte implantation procedure. Am J Sports Med 2010;38(6): 1259–71.

10. Arøen A, Løken S, Heir S, et al. Articular cartilage lesions in 993 consecutive knee arthroscopies. Am J Sports Med 2004;32:211–5.

11. Curl WW, Krome J, Gordon ES, et al. Cartilage injuries: a review of 31,516 knee arthroscopies. Arthroscopy 1997;13:456–60.

12. Widuchowski W, Widuchowski J, Trzaska T. Articular cartilage defects: study of 25,124 knee arthroscopies. Knee 2007;14:177–82.

13. D'Anchise R, Manta N, Prospero E, et al. Autologous implantation of chondrocytes on a solid collagen scaffold: clinical and histological outcomes after two years of follow-up. J Orthop Traumatol 2005;6:36–43.

14. Haddo O, Mahroof S, Higgs D, et al. The use of chondrogide membrane in autologous chondrocyte implantation. Knee 2004;11:51–5.

15. Micheli LJ, Moseley JB, Anderson AF, et al. Articular cartilage defects of the distal femur in children and adolescents: treatment with autologous chondrocyte implantation. J Pediatr Orthop 2006;26:455–60.

16. Heir S, Nerhus TK, Røtterud JH, et al. Focal cartilage defects in the knee impair quality of life as much as severe osteoarthritis: a comparison of knee injury and osteoarthritis outcome score in 4 patient categories scheduled for knee surgery. Am J Sports Med 2010;38:231–7.

17. Flachsmann R, Broom ND, Hardy AE, et al. Why is the adolescent joint particularly susceptible to osteochondral shear fracture? Clin Orthop Relat Res 2000;(381):212–21.

18. Detterline AJ, Goldberg S, Bach BR, et al. Treatment options for articular cartilage defects of the knee. Orthop Nurs 2005;24:361–6.

19. Gomoll AH, Farr J, Gillogly SD, et al. Surgical management of articular cartilage defects of the knee. J Bone Joint Surg Am 2010;92(14):2470–90.

20. Stuart MJ, Lubowitz JH. What, if any, are the indications for arthroscopic debridement of the osteoarthritic knee? Arthroscopy 2006;22:238.

21. Siparsky P, Ryzewicz M, Peterson B, et al. Arthroscopic treatment of osteoarthritis of the knee: are there any evidence-based indications? Clin Orthop Relat Res 2007;455:107–12.

22. Laupattarakasem W, Laopaiboon M, Laupattarakasem P, et al. Arthroscopic debridement for knee osteoarthritis. Cochrane Database Syst Rev 2008;1:CD005118.

23. Hunziker EB, Quinn TM. Surgical removal of articular cartilage leads to loss of chondrocytes from cartilage bordering the wound edge. J Bone Joint Surg Am 2003;85(Suppl 2):85–92.

24. Bedi A, Feeley BT, Williams RJ. Management of articular cartilage defects of the knee. J Bone Joint Surg Am 2010;92(4):994–1009.

25. Nehrer S, Minas T. Treatment of articular cartilage defects. Invest Radiol 2000;35:639.

26. Steinwachs MR, Guggi T, Kreuz PC. Marrow stimulation techniques. Injury 2008;39(Suppl 1):S26–31.

27. Tran-Khanh N, Hoemann CD, McKee MD, et al. Aged bovine chondrocytes display a diminished capacity to produce a collagen-rich, mechanically functional cartilage extracellular matrix. J Orthop Res 2005;23:1354–62.

28. Frisbie DD, Oxford JT, Southwood L, et al. Early events in cartilage repair after subchondral bone microfracture. Clin Orthop Relat Res 2003;407:215–27.

29. Bae DK, Yoon KH, Song SJ. Cartilage healing after microfracture in osteoarthritic knees. Arthroscopy 2006;22:367–74.

30. Steadman JR, Rodkey WG, Briggs KK. Microfracture to treat full-thickness chondral defects: surgical technique, rehabilitation, and outcomes. J Knee Surg 2002;15:170–6.

31. Harris JD, Siston RA, Pan X, et al. Autologous chondrocyte implantation: a systematic review. J Bone Joint Surg Am 2010;92(12):2220–33.

32. Kon E, Gobbi A, Filardo G, et al. Arthroscopic second-generation autologous chondrocyte implantation compared with microfracture for chondral lesions of the knee: prospective nonrandomized study at 5 years. Am J Sports Med 2009;37:33–41.

33. Mithoefer K, McAdams T, Williams RJ, et al. Clinical efficacy of the microfracture technique for articular cartilage repair in the knee: an evidence-based systematic analysis. Am J Sports Med 2009;37:2053–63.

34. Braune C, Rehart S, Kerschbaumer F, et al. Resorbable pin refixation of an osteochondral fracture of the lateral femoral condyle due to traumatic patellar dislocation: case management, follow-up and strategy in adolescents. Z Orthop Ihre Grenzgeb 2004;142(1):103–8 [in German].

35. Lüthje P, Nurmi-Lüthje I. Osteochondral fracture of the knee treated with bioabsorbable implants in two adolescents. Acta Orthop Belg 2008;74(2):249–54.

36. Jehan S, Loeffler MD, Pervez H. Osteochondral fracture of the lateral femoral condyle involving the entire weight bearing articular surface fixed with biodegradable screws. J Pak Med Assoc 2010;60(5):400–1.

37. Walsh SJ, Boyle MJ, Morganti V. Large osteochondral fractures of the lateral femoral condyle in the adolescent: outcome of bioabsorbable pin fixation. J Bone Joint Surg Am 2008;90(7):1473–8.

38. Camathias C, Festring JD, Gaston MS. Bioabsorbable lag screw fixation of knee osteochondritis dissecans in the skeletally immature. J Pediatr Orthop B 2011;20(2):74–80.

39. Dervin GF, Keene GC, Chissell HR. Biodegradable rods in adult osteochondritis dissecans of the knee. Clin Orthop Relat Res 1998;(356):213–21.

40. Sirlin CB, Boutin RD, Brossmann J, et al. Polydioxanone biodegradable pins in the knee: MR imaging. AJR Am J Roentgenol 2001;176(1):83–90.

41. Kerker JT, Leo AJ, Sgaglione NA. Cartilage repair: synthetics and scaffolds: basic science, surgical techniques, and clinical outcomes. Sports Med Arthrosc 2008;16(4):208–16.

42. Peterson L, Minas T, Brittberg M, et al. Treatment of osteochondritis dissecans of the knee with autologous chondrocyte transplantation: results at two to ten years. J Bone Joint Surg Am 2003;85(Suppl 2): 17–24.

43. Hangody L, Dobos J, Baló E, et al. Clinical experiences with autologous osteochondral mosaicplasty in an athletic population: a 17-year prospective multicenter study. Am J Sports Med 2010;38:1125–33.

44. Recht M, White LM, Winalski CS, et al. MR imaging of cartilage repair procedures. Skeletal Radiol 2003;32(4):185–200.

45. Kessler MW, Ackerman G, Dines JS, et al. Emerging technologies and fourth generation issues in cartilage repair. Sports Med Arthrosc 2008;16(4): 246–54.

46. Evans PJ, Miniaci A, Hurtig MB. Manual punch versus power harvesting of osteochondral grafts. Arthroscopy 2004;20:306–10.

47. Brittberg M, Lindahl A, Ohlsson C, et al. Treatment of deep cartilage defects in the knee with autologous chondrocyte transplantation. N Engl J Med 1994; 331:889–95.

48. Safran MR, Kim H, Zaffagnini S. The use of scaffolds in the management of articular cartilage injury. J Am Acad Orthop Surg 2008;16:306–11.

49. Tuan RS, Boland G, Tuli R. Adult mesenchymal stem cells and cell-based tissue engineering. Arthritis Res Ther 2003;5:32–45.

50. Daher RJ, Chahine NO, Greenberg AS, et al. New methods to diagnose and treat cartilage degeneration. Nat Rev Rheumatol 2009;5(11):599–607.

51. Saris DB, Vanlauwe J, Victor J, et al. Characterized chondrocyte implantation results in better structural repair when treating symptomatic cartilage defects of the knee in a randomized controlled trial versus microfracture. Am J Sports Med 2008;36:235–46.

52. Iwasa J, Engebretsen L, Shima Y, et al. Clinical application of scaffolds for cartilage tissue engineering. Knee Surg Sports Traumatol Arthrosc 2009;17(6):561–77.

53. Tuli R, Li W, Tuan RS. Current state of cartilage tissue engineering. Arthritis Res Ther 2003;5:235–8.

54. Zehbe R, Libera J, Gross U, et al. Short-term human chondrocyte culturing on oriented collagen coated gelatine scaffolds for cartilage replacement. Biomed Mater Eng 2005;15(6):445–54.

55. Kim HT, Zaffagnini S, Mizuno S, et al. A peek into the possible future of management of articular cartilage injuries: gene therapy and scaffolds for cartilage repair. J Orthop Sports Phys Ther 2006;36:765–73.

56. Bonaventure J, Kadhom N, Cohen-Solal L, et al. Re-expression of cartilage-specific genes by dedifferentiated human articular chondrocytes cultured in alginate beads. Exp Cell Res 1994;212:97–104.

57. Grande DA, Mason J, Light E, et al. Stem cells as platforms for delivery of genes to enhance cartilage repair. J Bone Joint Surg Am 2003;85(Suppl 2):111–6.

58. Peretti GM, Xu JW, Bonassar LJ, et al. Review of injectable cartilage engineering using fibrin gel in mice and swine models. Tissue Eng 2006;12(5):1151–68.

59. Kessler MW, Grande DA. Tissue engineering and cartilage. Organogenesis 2008;4:28–32.

60. Iwasaki N, Yamane ST, Majima T, et al. Feasibility of polysaccharide hybrid materials for scaffolds in cartilage tissue engineering: evaluation of chondrocyte adhesion to polyion complex fibers prepared from alginate and chitosan. Biomacromolecules 2004;5(3):828–33.

61. Sechriest VF, Miao YJ, Niyibizi C, et al. GAG-augmented polysaccharide hydrogel: a novel biocompatible and biodegradable material to support chondrogenesis. J Biomed Mater Res 2000;49(4):534–41.

62. Guo JF, Jourdian GW, MacCallum DK. Culture and growth characteristics of chondrocytes encapsulated in alginate beads. Connect Tissue Res 1989; 19:277–97.

63. Kujawa MJ, Caplan AI. Hyaluronic acid bonded to cell-culture surfaces stimulates chondrogenesis in stage 24 limb mesenchyme cell cultures. Dev Biol 1986;114:504–18.

64. Solchaga LA, Yoo JU, Lundberg M, et al. Hyaluronan-based polymers in the treatment of osteochondral defects. J Orthop Res 2000;18:773–80.

65. Nettles DL, Vail TP, Morgan MT, et al. Photocrosslinkable hyaluronan as a scaffold for articular cartilage repair. Ann Biomed Eng 2004;32(3):391–7.

66. Grigolo B, Lisignoli G, Piacentini A, et al. Evidence for redifferentiation of human chondrocytes grown on a hyaluronan-based biomaterial (HYAff 11): molecular, immunohistochemical and ultrastructural analysis. Biomaterials 2002;23(4):1187–95.

67. Brun P, Abatangelo G, Radice M, et al. Chondrocyte aggregation and reorganization into three-dimensional scaffolds. J Biomed Mater Res 1999; 46:337–46.

68. Marcacci M, Berruto M, Brocchetta D, et al. Articular cartilage engineering with Hyalograft C: 3-year clinical results. Clin Orthop Relat Res 2005;435:96–105.

69. Gobbi A, Kon E, Berruto M, et al. Patellofemoral full-thickness chondral defects treated with Hyalograft-C: a clinical, arthroscopic, and histologic review. Am J Sports Med 2006;34:1763–73.

70. Nehrer S, Domayer S, Dorotka R, et al. Three-year clinical outcome after chondrocyte transplantation using a hyaluronan matrix for cartilage repair. Eur J Radiol 2006;57(1):3–8.

71. Quinn TM, Schmid P, Hunziker EB, et al. Proteoglycan deposition around chondrocytes in agarose culture: construction of a physical and biological interface for mechanotransduction in cartilage. Biorheology 2002;39(1–2):27–37.

72. Ng KW, Wang CC, Mauck RL, et al. A layered agarose approach to fabricate depth-dependent inhomogeneity in chondrocyte-seeded constructs. J Orthop Res 2005;23(1):134–41.

73. Lee DA, Reisler T, Bader DL. Expansion of chondrocytes for tissue engineering in alginate beads enhances chondrocytic phenotype compared to conventional monolayer techniques. Acta Orthop Scand 2003;74(1):6–15.

74. Hoemann CD, Sun J, Légaré A, et al. Tissue engineering of cartilage using an injectable and adhesive chitosan-based cell-delivery vehicle. Osteoarthritis Cartilage 2005;13(4):318–29.

75. Li Z, Zhang M. Chitosan-alginate as scaffolding material for cartilage tissue engineering. J Biomed Mater Res A 2005;75(2):485–93.

76. Di Martino A, Sittinger M, Risbud MV. Chitosan: a versatile biopolymer for orthopaedic tissue-engineering. Biomaterials 2005;26:5983–90.

77. Shive MS, Hoemann CD, Restrepo A, et al. BST-cargel: in situ chondroinduction for cartilage repair. Operat Tech Orthop 2006;16(4):271–8.

78. Hoemann CD, Sun J, McKee MD, et al. Chitosanglycerol phosphate/blood implants elicit hyaline cartilage repair integrated with porous subchondral bone in microdrilled rabbit defects. Osteoarthritis Cartilage 2007;15(1):78–89.

79. Hoemann CD, Hurtig M, Rossomacha E, et al. Chitosan-glycerol phosphate/blood implants improve hyaline cartilage repair in ovine microfracture defects. J Bone Joint Surg Am 2005;87(12):2671–86.

80. Freyria AM, Cortial D, Ronzière MC, et al. Influence of medium composition, static and stirred conditions on the proliferation of and matrix protein expression of bovine articular chondrocytes cultured in a 3-D collagen scaffold. Biomaterials 2004;25(4):687–97.

81. Schulz RM, Zscharnack M, Hanisch I, et al. Cartilage tissue engineering by collagen matrix associated bone marrow derived mesenchymal stem cells. Biomed Mater Eng 2008;18(Suppl 1):S55–70.

82. Dorotka R, Windberger U, Macfelda K, et al. Repair of articular cartilage defects treated by microfracture and a three-dimensional collagen matrix. Biomaterials 2005;26(17):3617–29.

83. Zheng MH, Hinterkeuser K, Solomon K, et al. Collagen-derived biomaterials in bone and cartilage repair. Macromol Symp 2007;253:179–85.

84. Bartlett W, Skinner JA, Gooding CR, et al. Autologous chondrocyte implantation versus matrix-induced autologous chondrocyte implantation for osteochondral defects of the knee: a prospective, randomized study. J Bone Joint Surg Br 2005; 87(5):640–5.

85. Zeifang F, Oberle D, Nierhoff C, et al. Autologous chondrocyte implantation using the original periosteum-cover technique versus matrix-associated autologous chondrocyte implantation: a randomized clinical trial. Am J Sports Med 2010;38(5):924–33.

86. Chen G, Sato T, Ushida T, et al. The use of a novel PLGA fiber/collagen composite web as a scaffold for engineering of articular cartilage tissue with adjustable thickness. J Biomed Mater Res A 2003; 67(4):1170–80.

87. Munirah S, Kim SH, Ruszymah BH, et al. The use of fibrin and poly(lactic-co-glycolic acid) hybrid scaffold for articular cartilage tissue engineering: an in vivo analysis. Eur Cell Mater 2008;15:41–52.

88. Carmont MR, Carey-Smith R, Saithna A, et al. Delayed incorporation of a TruFit plug: perseverance is recommended. Arthroscopy 2009;25:810–4

89. Melton JT, Wilson AJ, Chapman-Sheath P, et al. TruFit CB bone plug: chondral repair, scaffold design, surgical technique and early experiences. Expert Rev Med Devices 2010;7:333–41.

90. Slivka MA, Leatherbury NC, Kieswetter K, et al. Porous, resorbable, fiber reinforced scaffolds tailored for articular cartilage repair. Tissue Eng 2001;7:767–80.

91. Niederauer GG, Slivka MA, Leatherbury NC, et al. Evaluation of multiphase implants for repair of focal osteochondral defects in goats. Biomaterials 2000; 21:2561–74.

92. Williams RJ, Gamradt SC. Articular cartilage repair using a resorbable matrix scaffold. Instr Course Lect 2008;57:563–71.

93. Dhollander AA, Liekens K, Almqvist KF, et al. A pilot study of the use of an osteochondral scaffold plug for cartilage repair in the knee and how to deal with early clinical failures. Arthroscopy 2012;28(2): 225–33.

94. Saithna AA, Carey-Smith R, Dhillon M, et al. Synthetic polymer scaffolds for repair of small articular cartilage defects of the knee: early clinical and radiological results. Presented at the British Orthopaedic Association Conference. Liverpool, September 16–19, 2008.

95. Davidson PA, Rivenburgh DW. Prospective evaluation of osteochondral defects in the knee treated with biodegradable scaffolds (SS-45). Presented at the 26th Annual Meeting of the Arthroscopic Association of North America Meeting, San Francisco, California, April 2007. Arthroscopy 2007;23(Suppl): e22–3.

Implantation of Orthobiologic, Biodegradable Scaffolds in Osteochondral Repair

James H.P. Hui, MBBS, FRCS, MD[a],*,
Kizher S. Buhary, MD, BE[a,b],
Ashwin Chowdhary, MBBS, D Orth, MS Orth, MRCS[a]

KEYWORDS

- Osteochondral repair • Scaffolds • Biologic
- Biodegradable

Osteochondral repair has been a therapeutic challenge owing to the complex biomechanical properties and poor healing capacity of articular cartilage.[1] Cartilage lesions have limited repair potential because of their avascular nature and lack of access to reparative and humoral factors that promote healing.[2] Full-thickness osteochondral defects that have access to the subchondral bone marrow cells, mesenchymal stem cells, growth factors, and cytokines are able to undergo repair, but fibrocartilage is deposited in place of hyaline articular cartilage.[3] A conservative approach to the treatment of the osteochondral defect significantly increases the risk of developing early osteoarthritis and functional disability.[4] Repair in weight-bearing joints such as the knee has been particularly challenging in pediatric patients who wish to resume levels of activity regardless of the pain, swelling, stiffness, or instability.

Current treatment methodologies include (1) microfracture,[5] (2) arthroscopic lavage and debridement,[6] (3) mosaicplasty,[7,8] (4) periosteal and perichondrial transplantation to full-thickness cartilage defects,[9] (5) autologous chondrocyte implantation,[10] and (6) cell-based and scaffold treatment.

Microfracture is a technique of bone marrow stimulation by creating perforations in the subchondral bone. This technique results in the migration of mesenchymal stem cells from the bone marrow to the site of the lesion, creating a clot.[11] The mesenchymal stem cells are then able to differentiate into fibrochondrocytes that participate in the repair of the chondral defect.[12] This technique, which is straightforward, is commonly used for the management of small chondral defects. However, studies have shown that the results are unsatisfactory in athletic[13] or elderly patients.[14]

Arthroscopic lavage and debridement can provide short-term relief. The goal of arthroscopic debridement and lavage is to reduce the inflammation and mechanical irritation within the joint. Debridement may include smoothening of the fibrillated articular surface, meniscal trimming, shaving of osteophytes, and removal of inflamed synovium. Joint lavage is thought to reduce synovitis and pain by washing fragments of cartilage and calcium phosphate crystals from the knee. Although these procedures have been reported to produce some temporary palliative effects, especially in older, low-demand patients, they are not a long-term solution.

No support or funds has been received for this work, and the authors have nothing to disclose.
[a] Division of Paediatric Orthopaedics, National University Hospital, 5, Lower Kent Ridge Road, Kent Ridge Wing 2, Level 3, 119074, Singapore
[b] Duke-NUS Graduate Medical School, Singapore
* Corresponding author.
E-mail address: James_hui@nuhs.edu.sg

Orthop Clin N Am 43 (2012) 255–261
doi:10.1016/j.ocl.2012.01.002

Resurfacing of the osteochondral defect is achieved via mosaicplasty. This technique involves the transfer of osteochondral plugs from less-weight-bearing surfaces of the medial and lateral condyles of the femur. Also known as autologous chondral mosaicplasty or osteoarticular transfer system (OTS), it provides several advantages such as the direct transplantation of hyaline cartilage, shorter rehabilitation duration, and being able to complete the technique in 1 surgery. Disadvantages include donor site morbidity, limited availability of grafts, and mismatch between donor and recipient graft sites, which could result in poor chondral integration.[15] Osteochondral allograft transplantation using either fresh, cryopreserved, or fresh-frozen allografts may overcome the disadvantage of donor site morbidity; however, this has a significant risk of immunologic rejection and disease transmission.[16]

Autologous chondrocyte implantation (ACI) has shown great promise for the treatment of full-thickness patellofemoral chondral defects. However, it presents some limitations: there is the need for general, or at least regional, anesthesia (to harvest the chondrocytes and transplant expanded cells) for 2-knee procedures. There is also the difficulty in obtaining an adequate number of chondrocytes, a slow rate of chondrocyte proliferation, and donor site morbidity.[17–19]

Cell-based therapies that involve either use of ACI or bone marrow–derived mesenchymal stem cells have evolved considerably. The use of biocompatible, biodegradable scaffolds onto which the cells are seeded has significant advantages such as an even distribution of cells and low donor site morbidity (because there is no need for periosteal harvesting or implantation, which also simplifies the technique).

The purpose of a scaffold is to act as a template to promote cellular interactions and formation of the extracellular matrix that provides the structural framework for the newly formed tissue. It is important that the scaffold, a temporary structure, mimics the physiologic conditions of the extracellular matrix because this affects the differentiation potential of the cells being seeded. There are certain requirements for a scaffold to be suitable for tissue engineering applications. It should be biocompatible, biodegradable, nonimmunogenic, and nontoxic. In addition, the structure of the scaffold (ie, both its macrostructural and microstructural properties) affects the potential for adequate cell survival, proliferation, growth, and organization within the scaffold construct. It also plays a significant role in gene expression and the modeling of cell shape.[20,21]

Porosity and interconnectivity of the scaffold play important roles in both in vitro and in vivo processes such as cell adhesion, growth, reorganization, and neovascularization.[22] Surface properties of the scaffold such as morphology, hydrophilicity, surface energy, and charge should also be considered because they influence the adhesion, migration, intracellular signaling, cell recruitment, and healing of the tissue-scaffold interface.[23] The mechanical strength of the scaffold should be similar to that of native tissue because this aids in withstanding the natural stresses and loads being applied, and prevents mechanical failure caused by premature loading of the native tissues.[24] This property is particularly critical in bone and cartilage tissue engineering scaffolds because these are weight-bearing tissues.

The integration of growth factors such as bone morphogenic proteins (BMPs) into the scaffold structure by means of structural entrapment or surface complexes (ionic or covalent bonding) has been widely used. Growth factors play an important role in guiding and controlling cellular behavior.[25] Novel methods are being explored, such as the use of growth factor–based microspheres[26] and bioactive microstructures (bioactive glass and ceramics)[27] to create scaffolds.

Natural and synthetic polymers have been used for cartilage regeneration. Synthetic polymers such as biodegradable and bioabsorbable polymers, polylactic-co-glycolic acid and polycaprolactone have been used for cartilage regeneration. Polyurethanes, polyhydroxyalkanoates, and polyphosphazene are some of the other synthetic polymers being investigated.[28] Natural polymers such as collagen, fibrin, and hyaluronic acid have also been used for the same purpose. Hydroxyapatite, calcium phosphates, and bioactive glasses are some of the inorganic materials that have been composited with polymers to significantly increase the bioactivity and mechanical properties of the scaffolds.[29,30]

Currently available treatment methodologies using scaffolds for osteochondral repair are (1) matrix-associated chondrocyte implantation (MACI), (2) hyaluronan-based scaffolds, and (3) tissue-engineered collagen scaffolds.

MACI

MACI is a technique that uses cultured autologous chondrocytes that are implanted onto a type I/III porcine collagen matrix. The cell seeding is done a few days before implantation. Results have shown expression of aggrecan, type II collagen, and S-100 with a 75% hyalinelike tissue at

6 months.[31] In a prospective randomized study comparing this technique with ACI, Bartlett and colleagues[32] found similar results, and 66% rated good to excellent scores on the International Cartilage Repair Scale (ICRS). Type I collagen has also been used as a matrix to support autologous chondrocytes.

By overcoming the need to harvest and implant a periosteal flap, MACI has a significant advantage compared with ACI in terms of graft site morbidity, and prevents dedifferentiation of the chondrocytes while being cultured in vitro. Arthroscopic techniques may be adopted for lesions that are accessible, thus reducing the hospital stay and postoperative complications such as periosteal hypertrophy[33] and arthrofibrosis.[34] In a multicenter study, Wood and colleagues[35] showed that open arthrotomy resulted in 26% of the procedure-related complications. Suture-free fixation has been explored using fibrin glue, which has shown a success rate of 88% in weight-bearing chondral defects of the femoral condyle.[36]

The efficacy of MACI was studied by Jones and colleagues[37] using animal models. They created 6-mm defects on the trochlea and medial femoral condyle that were treated with either MACI or unseeded, porcine-derived type I/III collagen membrane. At 10 weeks after surgery, arthroscopic assessment showed better fill, integration, and appearance in the study group. Magnetic resonance imaging (MRI) results were also consistent with MACI being superior to the control group. Immature cartilage and poor architectural constructs were seen in the control group.

Behrens and colleagues[38] reported on a 5-year follow-up of 34 patients treated with MACI. They found that these patients had a localized cartilage defect with a mean size of 4.1 cm^2. Lysholm-Gillquist, Meyer, and ICRS scores showed significant improvement in 11 patients (32.35%).

Trattnig and colleagues[39] used noninvasive cartilage-specific MRI to monitor 20 patients at sequential intervals following repair of cartilage defects using MACI. They found that an incomplete filling defect improved to a complete or less incomplete filling of the defect in 10 patients (50%). Within a year, 3 cases of cartilage hypertrophy returned to normal and integration with the native cartilage was complete in 10 patients. The signal intensity of the implanted cartilage was also found to be the same as that of the native cartilage in 13 patients (65%).

Bartlett and colleagues[40] studied the use of a sandwich technique using 2 MACI membranes on 8 patients (age range 18–46 years). The patients were subsequently assessed at 6 months and 1 year after surgery using the modified Cincinnati knee, the Stanmore functional rating, and the visual analog pain scores. Results showed that, within 6 months, all patients improved, with further improvement at the end of the first year. The clinical outcomes were also found to be good or excellent in 4 patients (50%) after 6 months and 1 year.

HYALURONAN-BASED SCAFFOLDS

Hyaluronic acid is a linear molecular mass polysaccharide that is commonly referred to as hyaluronan. Hyaluronan is a major component of the extracellular matrix of various connective tissues. It functions in providing structure as well as binding of bioactive molecules and behaves as a lubricant protecting articular cartilage surfaces.[41] It has been widely used in tissue engineering owing to its good biocompatibility, viscoelastic properties, nonimmunogenic properties, and ease of chain size manipulation. It also facilitates extracellular matrix remodeling via its interaction with cell surface receptors that promote the migration of cells.[42] Chow and colleagues[43] showed that, via cell surface receptor interactions with chondrocytes, hyaluronan allows the chondrocytes to maintain their native phenotype. Ehlers and colleagues[44] studied the effects of hyaluronic acid on the morphology and proliferation of human chondrocytes in primary cell culture. They concluded that hyaluronan stimulates the production of type II collagen and aggregan, and promotes cell proliferation. Hyaluronan has also been conjugated with alginate, chitosan, and fibrin gel matrices[45] and surface coated with type 1 collagen and fibronectin to facilitate cell attachment and tissue formation.[46]

Burdick and colleagues[47] used encapsulated porcine chondrocytes in photopolymerized hyaluronan hydrogels. They found that the cells maintained viability and were able to produce neocartilage within the porous network. Hyaluronan-derived polymers such as HYAFF7 and HYAFF11 have shown significant improvement in quality of healing of chondrocyte defects in vivo. In vitro studies have also shown that HYAFF11 3D scaffolds are able to reexpress their differentiated phenotype[48] and also reduce the expression and production of molecules involved in cartilage degeneration.[49] These scaffolds also have predictable degradation profiles that optimize the transition between newly formed and existing cellular matrices.[50] MRI and arthroscopic evaluation of chondral defects treated with Hyalograft C (autologous cells implanted onto an esterified hyaluronic acid scaffold) have shown regeneration of normal cartilage in more than 75% of patients. Gobbi and colleagues[51] studied 32 patellofemoral chondral lesions treated with Hyalograft C. They showed significant improvement in International Knee Documentation Committee (IKDC) scores in the course of a 2-year follow-up. MRI studies at 2 years' interval showed 71% to have normal cartilage. In 6 cases, second-look arthroscopies revealed the repaired surface to be near normal with biopsy samples characterized by hyalinelike appearance. The 3-year results of a multicenter clinical study by Maracacci and colleagues[52] showed similar results, with improved IKDC in 91.5% of patients. Preexisting cartilage defects had a mean size of 2.4 cm^2 and were Outerbridge grade III and IV. Normal or nearly normal postoperative arthroscopic evaluations were had by 96.4% of the patients in long-term follow-up. Histologic analysis showed hyalinelike cartilage in the lesion as early as 24 months after implantation. Subjective assessment also improved, with 76% and 88% of the patients having no pain or mobility problems, respectively.

Nehrer and colleagues[53] studied 53 patients with full-thickness chondral defects treated with Hyalograft C. They found a statistically significant increase in all knee scores of patients who were treated for the primary indications (young patient with stable joint, normal knee alignment, and isolated chondral defects with otherwise healthy adjacent cartilage). Patients who were treated for secondary indications as a salvage procedure showed poor results, with 9 of the 11 patients (81.8%) requiring total knee arthroplasty between 2 and 5 years after implantation.

Kon and colleagues[54] did a comparative study of autologous cartilage (hyaluronan-based scaffold) implantation and treatment with microfracture techniques for grade III and IV chondral lesions of the knee in 80 active patients (mean age, 29.8 years). In the course of a 5-year follow-up, they found significant improvement in IKDC in both groups. However, on return to sports, the scores remained stable after 5 years in the Hyalograft C group, whereas they worsened in the microfracture group. In a recent study, Kon and colleagues[55] showed that both techniques have similar success in returning to competitive-level sporting activity. Microfracture resulted in a faster recovery and return to competitive-level sporting activity compared with ACI. However, there was progressive clinical deterioration over time in the microfracture group, whereas ACI offered a more durable clinical outcome.

TISSUE ENGINEERED COLLAGEN SCAFFOLDS WITH MECHANICAL STIMULATION

In this technique, autologous chondrocytes are harvested and cultured in vitro and subsequently seeded onto bovine type I collagen scaffolds. These scaffolds have a honeycomb architecture and are subjected to mechanical stimulation with the use of bioreactors. The bioreactors use hydrostatic pressure to mechanically stimulate the chondrocytes for a period of 7 days.

Torzilli and colleagues[56] studied the role of mechanical load in the degradation in articular cartilage. Mature bovine articular cartilages were loaded with stresses for 3 days, followed by 3 days without stimulation. The investigators were able to see an increase in aggrean and a decrease in collagen loss. They concluded that a mechanical loading of the construct can slow the degradation of the extracellular matrix by chondrocytes when stimulated by interleukin 1 (IL-1). At the same time, excessive mechanical stimulation of the scaffold could lead to a significant increase in the hyaluronic acid catabolism by upregulation of IL-1 β mRNA levels.[57] A balance in the modulation of mechanical stimuli is hence imperative for optimal extracellular matrix formation.

Crawford and colleagues[58] used NeoCart, a tissue engineered collagen matrix seeded with autogenous chondrocytes, to treat 8 patients with full-thickness cartilage defects. They evaluated the outcome using IKDC scores, visual analog scale, range of motion, and cartilage-sensitive MRI over 24 months. They showed a significant decrease in pain scores compared with the preoperative measurements, and improved function and range of motion. MRI evaluation showed implanted cartilage stability, peripheral integration, organized cartilage formation, and 67% to 100% defect fill at 24 months.

SUMMARY

Millions of people around the world suffer from severe pain and disability as a result of cartilage trauma. The treatment of articular cartilage lesions is complicated. However, novel tissue engineering approaches seem to improve the outcome. Because using a tissue engineering approach is less invasive because of the lack of periosteal harvesting, it reduces surgical time, periosteal hypertrophy, and morbidity. Cell-based therapies using scaffolds have advantages compared with microfracture techniques, but the efficacy and cost-effectiveness need to be investigated. Second-generation cell-based therapies have lower morbidity and the ease of the technique is not significantly different from that of first-generation ACI techniques. Third-generation cell-based therapies such as the use of tissue-engineered scaffolds need to be studied in more detail. One of the challenges with using scaffold-based therapies is to control the accuracy and reproducibility of the scaffolds. Other procedural challenges include preparation of the chondral defect, scaffold integration, and also the long-term durability. Although preliminary studies have been promising, their effectiveness in the treatment of large chondral defects requires further long-term studies.

REFERENCES

1. Simon TM, Jackson DW. Articular cartilage: injury pathways and treatment options. Sports Med Arthrosc 2006;14:146–54.
2. Temenoff JS, Mikos AG. Review: tissue engineering for regeneration of articular cartilage. Biomaterials 2000;21:431–40.
3. Shapiro F, Koide S, Glimcher MJ. Cell origin and differentiation in the repair of full-thickness defects of articular cartilage. J Bone Joint Surg Am 1999;75:532–53.
4. Widuchowski W, Lukasik P, Kwiatkowski G, et al. Isolated full thickness chondral injuries. Prevalance and outcome of treatment. A retrospective study of 5233 knee arthroscopies. Acta Chir OrthopTraumatol Cech 2008;75:382–6.
5. Angel MJ, Razzano P, Grande DA. Defining the challenge – the basic science of articular cartilage repair and response to injury. Sports Med Arthrosc Rev 2003;11:168–81.
6. Jackson RW, Dietrichs C. The results of arthroscopic lavage and debridement of osteoarthritic knees based on the severity of degeneration: a 4- to 6-year symptomatic follow-up. Arthroscopy 2003;19:13–20.
7. Hangody L, Kish G, Karpati Z, et al. Mosaicplasty for the treatment of articular cartilage defects: application in clinical practice. Orthopedics 1998;21:751–6.
8. Kish G, Hangody L. A prospective, randomised comparison of autologous chondrocyte implantation versus mosaicplasty for osteochondral defects in the knee. J Bone Joint Surg Br 2004;86:619.
9. Carranza-Bencano A, Perez-Tinao M, Ballesteros-Vazquez P, et al. Comparative study of the reconstruction of articular cartilage defects with free costal perichondrial grafts and free tibial periosteal grafts: an experimental study on rabbits. Calcif Tissue Int 1999;65:402–7.
10. Nejadnik H, Hui JH, Feng Choong EP, et al. Autologous bone marrow–derived mesenchymal stem cells versus autologous chondrocyte implantation: an observational cohort study. Am J Sports Med 2010;38:1110.

11. Williams RJ 3rd, Harnly HW. Microfracture: indications, technique, and results. Instr Course Lect 2007;56:419–28.
12. Tran-Khanh N, Hoemann CD, McKee MD, et al. Aged bovine chondrocytes display a diminished capacity to produce a collagen-rich, mechanically functional cartilage extracellular matrix. J Orthop Res 2005;23:1354–62.
13. Mithoefer K, Williams RJ 3rd, Warren RF, et al. High-impact athletics after knee articular cartilage repair: a prospective evaluation of the microfracture technique. Am J Sports Med 2006;34:1413–8.
14. Kreuz PC, Erggelet C, Steinwachs MR, et al. Is microfracture of chondral defects in the knee associated with different results in patients aged 40 years or younger? Arthroscopy 2006;22:1180–6.
15. Hangody L, Vásárhelyi G, Hangody LR, et al. Autologous osteochondral grafting—technique and long-term results. Injury 2008;39(Suppl 1):S32–9.
16. Bugbee WD. Fresh osteochondral allografts. J Knee Surg 2002;15:191–5.
17. Bentley G, Biant LC, Carrington RW, et al. Randomised comparison of autologous chondrocyte implantation versus mosaicplasty for osteochondral defects in the knee. J Bone Joint Surg Br 2003;85(2):223–30.
18. Brittberg M, Lindahl A, Nilsson A, et al. Treatment of deep cartilage defects in the knee with autologous chondrocyte transplantation. N Engl J Med 1994;331(14):889–95.
19. Fu FH, Zurakowski D, Browne JE, et al. Autologous chondrocyte implantation versus debridement for treatment of full-thickness chondral defects of the knee: an observational cohort study with 3-year follow-up. Am J Sports Med 2005;33(11):1658–66.
20. Leong KF, Cheah CM, Chua CK. Solid freeform fabrication of three-dimensional scaffolds for engineering replacement tissues and organs. Biomaterials 2003;24:2363–78.
21. Karageorgiou V, Kaplan D. Porosity of 3D biomaterial scaffolds and osteogenesis. Biomaterials 2005;26:5474–91.
22. LeGeros RZ, LeGeros JP. Calcium phosphate biomaterials: preparation, properties, and biodegradation. In: Wise DL, Trantolo DJ, Altobelli DE, et al, editors. Encyclopedia handbook of biomaterials and bioengineering part A: materials, vol. 2. New York: Marcel Dekker; 1995. p. 1429–63.
23. Boyan BD, Hummert TW, Dean DD, et al. Role of material surfaces in regulating bone and cartilage cell response. Biomaterials 1996;17:137–46.
24. Carter DR, Blenman PR, Beaupré GS. Correlations between mechanical stress history and tissue differentiation in initial fracture healing. J Orthop Res 1988;6:736–48.
25. Schmidt MB, Chen EH, Lynch SE. A review of the effects of insulin-like growth factor and platelet

derived growth factor on in vivo cartilage healing and repair. Osteoarthr Cartil 2006;14:403–12.

26. Schrier J, Fink B, Rodgers J, et al. Effect of a freeze dried CMC/PLGA microsphere matrix of rhBMP-2 on bone healing. AAPS PharmSciTech 2001;2:73–80.

27. Hench LL. Bioceramics. J Am Ceram Soc 1998;81: 1705–28.

28. Vinatier C, Mrugala D, Jorgensen C, et al. Cartilage engineering: a crucial combination of cells, biomaterials and biofactors. Trends Biotechnol 2009;27: 307–14.

29. Rezwan K, Chen QZ, Blaker JJ, et al. Biodegradable and inorganic composite scaffolds for bone tissue engineering. Biomaterials 2006;27:3413–31.

30. Habraken WJ, Wolke JG, Jansen JA. Ceramic composites as matrices and scaffolds for drug delivery in tissue engineering. Adv Drug Deliv Rev 2007;59:234–48.

31. Zheng MH, Willers C, Kirilak L, et al. (MACI): biological and histological assessment. Tissue Eng 2007; 13:737–46.

32. Muller-Rath R, Gavenis K, Andereya S, et al. A novel rat tail collagen type-I gel for the cultivation of human articular chondrocytes in low cell density. Int J Artif Organs 2007;30:1057–67.

33. Minas T. Autologous chondrocyte implantation for focal chondral defects of the knee. Clin Orthop Relat Res 2001;391(Suppl):S349–61.

34. Micheli LJ, Browne JE, Erggelet C, et al. Autologous chondrocyte implantation of the knee: multicenter experience and minimum 3-year follow-up. Clin J Sport Med 2001;11:223–8.

35. Wood JJ, Malek MA, Frassica FJ, et al. Autologous cultured chondrocytes: adverse events reported to the United States Food and Drug Administration. J Bone Joint Surg Am 2006;88:503–7.

36. Marlovits S, Striessnig G, Kutscha-Lissberg F, et al. Early postoperative adherence of matrix-induced autologous chondrocyte implantation for the treatment of full-thickness cartilage defects of the femoral condyle. Knee Surg Sports Traumatol Arthrosc 2005;13:451–7.

37. Jones CW, Willers C, Keogh A, et al. Matrix-induced autologous chondrocyte implantation in sheep: objective assessments including confocal arthroscopy. J Orthop Res 2008;26:292–303.

38. Behrens P, Bitter T, Kurz B, et al. Matrix-associated autologous chondrocyte transplantation/implantation (MACT/MACI)—5-year follow-up. Knee 2006; 13:194–202.

39. Trattnig S, Ba-Ssalamah A, Pinker K, et al. Matrix-based autologous chondrocyte implantation for cartilage repair: noninvasive monitoring by high-resolution magnetic resonance imaging. Magn Reson Imaging 2005;23:451–7.

40. Bartlett W, Gooding CR, Carrington RW, et al. Autologous chondrocyte implantation at the knee using a bilayer collagen membrane with bone graft. A preliminary report. J Bone Joint Surg Br 2005;87: 330–2.

41. Campoccia D, Doherty P, Radice M, et al. Semisynthetic resorbable materials from hyaluronan esterification. Biomaterials 1998;19:2101–27.

42. Allison DD, Grande-Allen KJ. Review. Hyaluronan: a powerful tissue engineering tool. Tissue Eng 2006;12:2131–40.

43. Chow G, Knudson CB, Homandberg G, et al. Increased expression of CD44 in bovine articular chondrocytes by catabolic cellular mediators. J Biol Chem 1995;270:27734–41.

44. Ehlers EM, Behrens P, Wünsch L, et al. Effects of hyaluronic acid on the morphology and proliferation of human chondrocytes in primary cell culture. Ann Anat 2001;183:13–7.

45. Lindenhayn K, Perka C, Spitzer RS, et al. Retention of hyaluronic acid in alginate beads: aspects for in vitro cartilage engineering. J Biomed Mater Res 1999;44:149–55.

46. Ramamurthi A, Vesely I. Smooth muscle cell adhesion on crosslinked hyaluronan gels. J Biomed Mater Res 2002;60:195–205.

47. Burdick JA, Chung C, Jia X, et al. Controlled degradation and mechanical behavior of photopolymerized hyaluronic acid networks. Biomacromolecules 2004;6:386–91.

48. Grigolo B, Lisignoli G, Piacentini A, et al. Evidence for redifferentiation of human chondrocytes grown on a hyaluronan-based biomaterial (HYAFF(R)11): molecular, immunohistochemical and ultrastructural analysis. Biomaterials 2002;23:1187–95.

49. Grigolo B, De Franceschi L, Roseti L, et al. Down regulation of degenerative cartilage molecules in chondrocytes grown on a hyaluronan-based scaffold. Biomaterials 2005;26:5668–76.

50. Kang JY, Chung CW, Sung JH, et al. Novel porous matrix of hyaluronic acid for the three-dimensional culture of chondrocytes. Int J Pharm 2009;369: 114–20.

51. Gobbi A, Kon E, Berruto M, et al. Patellofemoral full-thickness chondral defects treated with Hyalograft-C: a clinical, arthroscopic, and histologic review. Am J Sports Med 2006;34:1763–73.

52. Marcacci M, Berruto M, Brocchetta D, et al. Articular cartilage engineering with Hyalograft C: 3-year clinical results. Clin Orthop Relat Res 2005;435: 96–105.

53. Nehrer S, Dorotka R, Domayer S, et al. Treatment of full-thickness chondral defects with Hyalograft C in the knee: a prospective clinical case series with 2 to 7 years' follow-up. Am J Sports Med 2009; 37(Suppl 1):81S–7S.

54. Kon E, Gobbi A, Filardo G, et al. Arthroscopic second-generation autologous chondrocyte implantation compared with microfracture for chondral

lesions of the knee: prospective nonrandomized study at 5 years. Am J Sports Med 2009;37:33–41.

55. Kon E, Filardo G, Berruto M, et al. Articular cartilage treatment in high-level male soccer players: a prospective comparative study of arthroscopic second-generation autologous chondrocyte implantation versus microfracture. Am J Sports Med 2011;39(12): 2549–57.

56. Torzilli PA, Bhargava M, Park S, et al. Mechanical load inhibits IL-1 induced matrix degradation in articular cartilage. Osteoarthr Cartil 2010;18(1): 97–105.

57. Tanimoto K, Kitamura R, Tanne Y, et al. Modulation of hyaluronan catabolism in chondrocytes by mechanical stimuli. J Biomed Mater Res A 2010;93(1):373–80.

58. Crawford DC, Heveran CM, Cannon WD Jr, et al. An autologous cartilage tissue implant NeoCart for treatment of grade III chondral injury to the distal femur: prospective clinical safety trial at 2 years. Am J Sports Med 2009;39:1334–43.

Index

Note: Page numbers of article titles are in **boldface** type.

A

Age
  as factor in OCD, 237
Aging
  of articular cartilage, 190
Arthritis
  in children, **213–225**. *See also* Juvenile idiopathic
    arthritis (JIA)
  enthesis-related
    in children, 214
      pathogenesis of, 216
  juvenile idiopathic, **213–225**. *See also* Juvenile
    idiopathic arthritis (JIA)
  oligoarticular/polyarticular
    in children
      pathogenesis of, 215
  psoriatic
    in children, 214–215
      pathogenesis of, 214
  systemic idiopathic
    in children
      pathogenesis of, 215–216
  undifferentiated
    in children, 215
Arthropathy
  joint-related
    exercise effects on, 192–193
Arthroscopic BMCD transplantation
  in "one step" treatment of OCD in knee, 239–240
Articular cartilage
  aging of, 190
  cartilage extracellular matrix, 188
  cartilage matrix compartmentalization in, 190
  chondrons in, 188
  collagens in, 188–189
  described, 188, 245
  development of, **155–171**
    articular-epiphyseal cartilage, 156–157
    chondrogenesis, 158–162. *See also*
      Chondrogenesis, of articular cartilage
    endochondral ossification of, 162–165
      cartilage matrix modeling during, 165–167
      molecular factors in, 162–165
        bone morphogenetic proteins, 164
        TGF-β, 164
        Wnt family, 164–165
  exercise effects on, **187–199**. *See also* Exercise,
    articular cartilage effects of
  growth of

    during chondrogenesis, 160
  imaging in evaluation of
    in JIA, 222–223
  injuries of
    prevalence of, 245–246
    repair of. *See also* Cartilage engineering,
      scaffolds for
      bone marrow–stimulating techniques in,
        246–247
      nonoperative therapy in, 246
      nonreparative/nonrestorative procedures
        in, 246
      restorative techniques in, 247–248
      tissue engineering/scaffold in, 248–251
  mature, 157–158
  noncollagenous proteins in, 189–190
  proteoglycans in, 189
  repair of
    limited capability in, 245–246
  role of, 187
  structure and function of, 155–156
Articular-epiphyseal cartilage
  development of, 156–157

B

Biodegradable scaffolds
  in articular cartilage injury repair, 251
BMCD transplantation. *See* Bone marrow–derived
  cell (BMDC) transplantation
BMP. *See* Bone morphogenetic proteins (BMP)
Bone
  structural and functional maturation of
    during postnatal development and growth
      studies of, **173–185**. *See also* Distal femoral
        cartilage and bone, structural and
        functional maturation of, during
        postnatal development and growth,
        studies of
Bone marrow
  imaging in evaluation of
    in JIA, 222–223
Bone marrow aspiration
  in "one step" treatment of OCD in knee, 239
Bone marrow concentration
  in "one step" treatment of OCD in knee, 239
Bone marrow–derived cell (BMDC) transplantation
  arthroscopic
    in "one step" treatment of OCD in knee,
      239–240

Orthop Clin N Am 43 (2012) 263–267
doi:10.1016/S0030-5898(12)00020-X

orthopedic.theclinics.com

Moving?

Make sure your subscription moves with you!

To notify us of your new address, find your **Clinics Account Number** (located on your mailing label above your name), and contact customer service at:

Email: journalscustomerservice-usa@elsevier.com

800-654-2452 (subscribers in the U.S. & Canada)
314-447-8871 (subscribers outside of the U.S. & Canada)

Fax number: 314-447-8029

Elsevier Health Sciences Division
Subscription Customer Service
3251 Riverport Lane
Maryland Heights, MO 63043

*To ensure uninterrupted delivery of your subscription, please notify us at least 4 weeks in advance of move.